Antiepileptic Drugs

Antiepileptic Drugs

A Clinician's Manual

Second Edition

Ali A. Asadi-Pooya, MD

Associate Professor of Epileptology
Director, Shiraz Comprehensive Epilepsy Center
Department of Neurology
Shiraz University of Medical Sciences
Shiraz, Iran

Jefferson Comprehensive Epilepsy Center
Department of Neurology
Thomas Jefferson University
Philadelphia, PA

Michael R. Sperling, MD

Baldwin Keyes Professor of Neurology
Vice Chair for Clinical Affairs
Director, Jefferson Comprehensive Epilepsy Center
Department of Neurology
Thomas Jefferson University
Philadelphia, PA

OXFORD
UNIVERSITY PRESS

OXFORD
UNIVERSITY PRESS

Oxford University Press is a department of the University of Oxford. It furthers
the University's objective of excellence in research, scholarship, and education
by publishing worldwide. Oxford is a registered trademark of Oxford University
Press in the UK and certain other countries.

Published in the United States of America by Oxford University Press
198 Madison Avenue, New York, NY 10016, United States of America.

Library of Congress Cataloging-in-Publication Data
Names: Asadi-Pooya, Ali A., 1973–, author. | Sperling, Michael R., author.
Title: Antiepileptic drugs : a clinician's manual / Ali A. Asadi-Pooya, Michael R. Sperling.
Description: Second edition. | New York, NY : Oxford University Press, 2016.
| Includes bibliographical references and index.
Identifiers: LCCN 2015037223 | ISBN 9780190214968 (paperback : alk. paper)
Subjects: | MESH: Anticonvulsants—therapeutic use—Handbooks. |
Epilepsy—drug therapy—Handbooks.
Classification: LCC RM322 | NLM QV 39 | DDC 615/.784—dc23
LC record available at http://lccn.loc.gov/2015037223

9 8 7 6 5 4 3 2 1

Printed in Canada

Contents

CONTENTS

vi

Chapter 1

Diagnosis and Evaluation of Patients With Seizures

Approximately 10% of the general population will experience at least one seizure within their lifetimes in most Western countries, and even higher rates are observed in developing countries. However, not all individuals go on to develop epilepsy, which is characterized by recurring epileptic seizures. An *epileptic seizure* is the transient occurrence of signs or symptoms due to abnormal excessive, hypersynchronous firing of neurons in the brain. The new practical clinical definition of epilepsy proposed by the International League Against Epilepsy (ILAE) considers epilepsy to be a disease of the brain defined by any of the following conditions: (1) at least two unprovoked (or reflex) seizures occurring >24 hours apart; (2) one unprovoked (or reflex) seizure and a probability of further seizures similar to the general recurrence risk (at least 60%) after two unprovoked seizures, occurring over the next 10 years; and (3) diagnosis of an epilepsy syndrome (Fisher et al., 2014). Epilepsy may be due to genetic causes (possessing an inherited trait to have seizures), brain tumors, infections (meningitis or encephalitis), brain trauma, stroke, developmental anomalies (eg, cortical dysplasia), malformations (tuberous sclerosis, neurofibromatosis), vascular malformations (arteriovenous malformations), and other causes.

To properly diagnose "epilepsy" a physician must do more than simply establish that recurrent seizures have occurred or are highly likely to occur after the first one. It is important that an attempt be made to diagnose a specific *epilepsy syndrome*. This syndrome forms the basis for the health provider to decide on therapy. The syndrome reflects the constellation of historical features, symptoms, signs, and laboratory test results that define a distinct condition. Hence, the syndromic diagnosis involves more than just the seizure type; frontal lobe seizures, for instance, do not constitute a syndrome. In contrast, benign Rolandic epilepsy of childhood does constitute a distinct syndrome, with its characteristic etiology, natural history, seizure type, developmental history, neurological examination, and electroencephalogram (EEG) abnormality (Box 1.1). An *idiopathic (genetic) epilepsy syndrome* is the direct result of a known or inferred genetic defect(s). Seizures are the core symptom of the disorder. It appears at a specific age (age dependent) with no underlying structural brain lesions or related neurological abnormalities. Examples of idiopathic (genetic) syndromes include benign Rolandic epilepsy of childhood, childhood absence epilepsy, and juvenile myoclonic epilepsy. A *symptomatic (structural-metabolic) epilepsy syndrome* is the result of an identifiable structural or metabolic lesion of the

Box 1.1 Important Epilepsy Syndromes Based on the International League Against Epilepsy (ILAE) Classification

General Classification	Syndrome	Description
Idiopathic (genetic) generalized epilepsies	Childhood and juvenile absence epilepsies	Childhood absence epilepsy (pyknolepsy) occurs in children of school age (peak manifestation age 6 to 7 years), with a strong genetic predisposition in otherwise normal children. It is characterized by very frequent (several to many per day) absences. The EEG reveals bilateral usually 3 Hz, synchronous spike waves or polyspikes and waves, on a normal background activity. During adolescence, generalized tonic-clonic seizures often develop.
		Juvenile absence epilepsy develops insidiously in physically and mentally healthy adolescents. Age at onset is usually between 10 and 17 years (peak between 10 and 12 years). Because the frequency of the absences is low and the symptoms are relatively trivial, the disorder may go unnoticed until generalized tonic-clonic seizures appear.
	Juvenile myoclonic epilepsy	Juvenile myoclonic epilepsy typically appears in the second decade of life. The age of onset often ranges from 8 to 24 years, with peak onset between 14 and 16 years. It is characterized by myoclonic seizures, associated at times with generalized tonic-clonic seizures or absence seizures.
	Epilepsy with myoclonic-astatic seizures (Doose syndrome)	Prior to the onset of myoclonic-astatic seizures, most affected children show normal development. The seizures usually begin between 2 and 5 years of age. The first seizure is most often a generalized tonic-clonic seizure and rarely a myoclonic, astatic, myoclonic-astatic, or absence seizure. Drop attacks may result from pure astatic, myoclonic-astatic, or atypical absence seizures.
Epileptic encephalopathies (in which the epileptiform abnormalities may contribute to progressive dysfunction)	West syndrome	West syndrome is an age-dependent epilepsy syndrome that comprises a triad of epileptic spasms in clusters, mental retardation, and diffuse and profound paroxysmal EEG abnormalities in infancy.

(continued)

Box 1.1 (Continued)

General Classification	Syndrome	Description
	Severe myoclonic epilepsy in infancy (Dravet syndrome)	Severe myoclonic epilepsy begins during the first year of life. Development is normal prior to the onset of seizures. Affected infants develop either generalized or unilateral clonic seizures without prodromal signs. Myoclonic jerks, absence seizures, and partial seizures usually appear later. The occurrence of status epilepticus is frequent. Psychomotor retardation and other neurological deficits occur in affected children.
	Lennox-Gastaut syndrome	The Lennox-Gastaut syndrome is, with rare exception, a condition of children. It is characterized by the clinical triad of multiple types of seizures, including especially atypical absences and tonic and atonic seizures, diffuse slow spikes-and-waves and/or generalized paroxysmal fast activity on an abnormal background activity in EEG, and mental retardation (mental retardation is not a mandatory element).
	Landau-Kleffner syndrome	Age of onset for Landau-Kleffner syndrome ranges from 3 to 8 years, and boys are more frequently affected than girls. Acquired aphasia (verbal auditory agnosia) is the more prominent feature, because seizures are present in only 70% to 80% of the patients.
Progressive myoclonic epilepsies		Include: ceroid lipofuscinosis, sialidosis, Lafora disease, Unverricht-Lundborg disease, neuroaxonal dystrophy, MERRF, and dentatorubropallidoluysian atrophy.
Idiopathic (genetic) focal epilepsies	BECTS (Rolandic epilepsy)	Benign epilepsy of childhood with centrotemporal spikes (BECTS) has five criteria for the diagnosis: (1) onset between the ages of 2 and 13 years; (2) absence of neurological or intellectual deficit before the onset; (3) partial seizures with motor signs, frequently associated with somatosensory symptoms or precipitated by sleep; (4) a spike focus located in the centrotemporal (rolandic) area with normal background activity on the interictal EEG; and (5) spontaneous remission during adolescence.
	Benign occipital epilepsies	Panayiotopoulos syndrome is best described as early-onset benign childhood seizure susceptibility syndrome with mainly autonomic seizures (e.g., ictus emeticus) and autonomic status epilepticus.

(continued)

Box 1.1 (Continued)

General Classification	Syndrome	Description
		The cardinal features of late-onset childhood occipital epilepsy (Gastaut type) are visual seizures predominantly manifested with elementary visual hallucinations, blindness, or both. They are usually frequent and diurnal, and they usually last from seconds to 1 to 3 minutes.
Symptomatic (or probably symptomatic) focal epilepsies	Limbic epilepsies	Include: mesial temporal lobe epilepsy with hippocampal sclerosis and mesial temporal lobe epilepsy defined by specific etiologies.
	Neocortical epilepsies	Include: Rasmussen syndrome, hemiconvulsion-hemiplegia syndrome, and migrating partial seizures of early infancy.

Note: Febrile seizures (febrile convulsions) are the most common convulsive events in human experience. Febrile seizures can be categorized as either "simple" (generalized tonic-clonic seizure, duration less than 15 minutes and without recurrence within 24 hours) or "complex" (focal seizure, lasting more than 15 minutes or occurring in a cluster of 2 or more convulsions within 24 hours). Febrile seizures are generally benign and only 2% to 3% of children will later develop epilepsy, primarily those who have complex febrile seizures.

From the International League Against Epilepsy website (http://www.ilae-epilepsy.org/visitors/centre/ctf/) with minor modifications.

brain, such as cerebral infarction, brain tumor, cortical dysplasia, or ceroid lipo-fuscinosis. A *probable symptomatic (unknown) epilepsy syndrome* is synonymous with cryptogenic epilepsy, and this term defines syndromes that are believed to be symptomatic, but no etiology has been identified (Berg et al., 2010; Blume et al., 2001; Engel, 2006).

The International League Against Epilepsy (ILAE) classifies seizures as either partial (focal) or generalized. Focal epileptic seizures are conceptualized as originating within networks limited to one hemisphere. These may be discretely localized or more widely distributed. Generalized epileptic seizures are conceptualized as originating at some point within, and rapidly engaging, bilaterally distributed networks (Berg et al., 2010).

Definitions for the major seizure types include the following (Blume et al., 2001):

Motor Seizures

- Tonic: A sustained increase in muscle contraction lasting a few seconds to a few minutes.
- Clonic: Myoclonus that is regularly repetitive, involves the same muscle groups, usually at a starting frequency of 2–3 jerks per second, and is prolonged.

- Tonic-clonic: A sequence consisting of a tonic phase followed by a clonic phase. Variants such as clonic-tonic-clonic may be seen.
- Myoclonic: Sudden, brief (<100 milliseconds) involuntary single or multiple contraction(s) of muscles(s) or muscle groups of variable topography (axial, proximal limb, distal limb).
- Atonic: Sudden loss or diminution of muscle tone without apparent preceding myoclonic or tonic event lasting ≥1 to 2 seconds; involving head, trunk, jaw, or limb musculature. Synonym: drop attack.
- Astatic: Loss of erect posture that results from an atonic, myoclonic, or tonic mechanism. Synonym: drop attack.
- Epileptic spasm (formerly infantile spasm): A sudden flexion, extension, or mixed extension-flexion of predominantly proximal and truncal muscles that is usually more sustained than a myoclonic movement but not so sustained as a tonic seizure (ie, 1 second). Limited forms may occur: grimacing, head nodding. Epileptic spasms frequently occur in clusters.
- Automatism: The ILAE defines automatism as more or less coordinated, often repetitive, motor activity usually occurring when cognition is impaired and for which the subject is usually amnesic. This often resembles a voluntary movement and may consist of an inappropriate continuation of ongoing preictal motor activity.

Nonmotor Seizures

- Aura: A subjective phenomenon that precedes an observable seizure and for which memory is retained afterward. This may consist of a sensory, psychic, autonomic, or other nonspecific subjective symptoms. Because of retrograde amnesia, some patients may not recall the experience of an aura.
- Sensory seizure: A perceptual experience not produced by stimuli from the external world.
- Dyscognitive seizures: Events in which disturbance of cognition is the prominent or most apparent feature, with alterations in perception, attention, emotion, memory, or execution function.

Seizure types based on the latest proposed ILAE classification scheme include the following (Berg et al., 2010; Blume et al., 2001):

Generalized Seizures

- Tonic-clonic seizures
- Clonic seizures
- Absence seizures
  - Typical
  - Atypical
  - Absence with special features
    - Myoclonic-absence
    - Eyelid myoclonia

- Tonic seizures
- Spasms
- Myoclonic seizures
  - Myoclonic
  - Myoclonic-atonic
  - Myoclonic-tonic
- Atonic seizures
- Reflex seizures in generalized epilepsy syndromes

Focal Seizures

- Focal sensory seizures
  - With elementary sensory symptoms (unformed phenomena from one primary sensory modality, eg, somatosensory, visual, auditory, olfactory, gustatory, epigastric, or cephalic)
  - With experiential sensory symptoms (eg, temporo-parieto-occipital junction seizures)
- Focal motor seizures
  - With elementary clonic motor signs
  - With asymmetrical tonic motor seizures (eg, supplementary motor seizures)
  - With typical (temporal lobe) automatisms (eg, mesial temporal lobe seizures)
  - With hyperkinetic automatisms
  - With focal negative myoclonus
  - With inhibitory motor seizures
- Gelastic seizures
- Hemiclonic seizures
- Secondarily generalized seizures
- Reflex seizures in focal epilepsy syndromes

Continuous Seizure Types

- Generalized status epilepticus
  - Generalized tonic-clonic status epilepticus
  - Clonic status epilepticus
  - Tonic status epilepticus
  - Absence status epilepticus
  - Myoclonic status epilepticus
- Focal status epilepticus
  - Epilepsia partialis continua
  - Aura continua
  - Limbic status epilepticus (psychomotor status)
  - Hemiconvulsive status with hemiparesis

Evaluation of a Patient Suspected to Have an Epileptic Seizure

Diagnosis of Epilepsy

Epilepsy is a clinical diagnosis. Unless one happens to observe a seizure while recording the EEG, which is a rare event in general clinical practice, the diagnosis relies on the judgment of a physician or other health-care provider. This judgment ultimately rests on the history provided by the patient and others. Therefore, careful attention must be paid when obtaining the relevant historical details, and one must systematically establish whether a seizure has really occurred and what type of seizure it was. Hence, when evaluating a patient with a possible seizure disorder, one must first determine whether seizures have truly occurred or whether a disorder exists that mimics epilepsy. The differential diagnosis includes convulsive or nonconvulsive syncope, transient ischemic attacks, complicated migraines, hypoglycemia, panic attacks, sleep disorders, Méniére's disease, psychogenic non-epileptic seizures, and movement disorders. In children, one must also consider night terrors, breath-holding spells, colic, and tics. An incorrect diagnosis may have many negative consequences. If the diagnosis is that of a seizure, one must then determine whether the seizure is primary and arises from the brain, or secondary, due to transient ischemia from a primary cardiovascular disorder. Symptoms that precede the seizure or occur when it begins, as well as behaviors exhibited during seizures, offer clues as to the type of seizure and therefore the diagnosis (Asadi-Pooya & Emami, 2012; Asadi-Pooya, Emami, & Sperling, 2013).

Neurologists and other physicians occasionally must distinguish seizures from syncope. Syncope is the impairment of cardiovascular autonomic control, which results in gradual failure of cerebral perfusion. Syncope is often associated with pallor, cold and clammy skin, and perhaps electrocardiographic or blood pressure abnormalities. However, syncope may be associated with one or more jerks at the onset of loss of consciousness or even convulsive activity, leading to ambiguity in diagnosis (Asadi-Pooya et al., 2011). With generalized tonic-clonic seizures, patients typically have increased tone (tonic phase) followed by clonic repetitive jerks associated with labored respiration, flushed color, and incontinence or tongue biting. To differentiate epileptic seizures from other possible diagnoses, details about timing may also be helpful. Most complex partial seizures last from 30 seconds to 3 minutes, while movement disorders and panic attacks may last longer. Breath-holding spells and panic attacks typically have an inciting event. Sleep state may help distinguish between different diagnoses, because some occur only while a person is asleep and others do not. One must also consider whether there are risk factors that would heighten suspicion for seizures, such as developmental delay, antecedent brain injury, preexisting neurological impairments, family history of epilepsy, and so forth. Therefore, history is the key step in diagnosing epileptic seizures.

History

The key element in making the correct diagnosis of an epilepsy syndrome is obtaining a detailed clinical history. This includes:

- **Seizure description:** It is critical that a history be obtained from the patient as well as a witness. You should begin by asking the patient and observer to describe in detail the events that occurred before, during, and after the seizure. While individuals may have more than one type of seizure, seizures are typically stereotyped. Other useful clues include sleep/wake cycle, concurrent symptoms (eg, fever, headache, vomiting, etc.), precipitating factors, other comorbidities, and family history of epilepsy.
- **Risk factors for seizures:** It is important to know the risk factors for seizures. However, while there are many risk factors for epilepsy (eg, perinatal insults, developmental delay, head trauma, infections, genetic tendency, acquired brain lesions), many patients have no obvious etiology.
- **A complete history:** past history, family, and social history can be useful.

Physical Examination

Most individuals with epilepsy have a relatively normal general and neurological examination unless they have an underlying significant focal structural abnormality. Usually, if deficits are present, they are subtle and often appear solely as a variety of cognitive and language deficits. It is important to evaluate for skin lesions and other congenital abnormalities, such as adenoma sebaceum associated with tuberous sclerosis. It is also helpful to examine for body hemiatrophy. On occasion, hyperventilation in the office will trigger an absence seizure in individuals with generalized epilepsy.

Electroencephalography

The EEG is a test that evaluates the electrical activity of the brain. The EEG provides information concerning the presence or absence of abnormal electrical activity, as well as information that aids in classification of the disorder and location of the seizure focus. The EEG should be recorded during wakefulness and sleep to optimize chances of detecting an abnormality. Activation procedures such as photic stimulation and hyperventilation may help elicit epileptiform activity as well.

A normal EEG does not rule out the clinical diagnosis of epileptic seizures, and for approximately 50% of patients with epilepsy, a single EEG will be normal. If the suspicion of epilepsy is high, additional EEG recording after sleep deprivation or an ambulatory 24-hour EEG may improve the yield to approximately 90%.

Laboratory Tests and Neuroimaging

These studies are performed to determine the cause of a newly diagnosed seizure disorder. They may include electrolyte and liver function tests, toxicology screen, and chemistry panel if a patient is seen acutely after a seizure. Lumbar puncture is performed only if an infection or malignancy is suspected.

Magnetic resonance imaging (MRI) is the most important test for many patients. It is appropriate to obtain an MRI scan to assess for a structural lesion if the epilepsy is not believed to be due to a genetic cause (eg, childhood absence epilepsy, juvenile myoclonic epilepsy, benign Rolandic epilepsy, etc.). An MRI is preferable to a computed tomography scan because it has greater sensitivity. It detects macroscopic structural lesions, such as tumors, encephalomalacia, cortical dysplasias, and mesial temporal sclerosis (atrophy of the hippocampus). The latter abnormality is the most common finding in individuals with medial temporal lobe epilepsy, a common type of epilepsy characterized by recurrent complex partial seizures. Coronal sections using FLAIR sequences and coronal thin-section sequences using T1 sequences optimally display mesial temporal sclerosis. An MRI scan is recommended after a first seizure in anyone who does not have a clear genetic cause for the seizure. In particular, it is required if a patient had a focal seizure, a focal neurological deficit, persistently altered mental status, a history of trauma, persistent headache, a history of cancer or anticoagulation therapy, suspected infection, HIV infection, and (in children) cognitive or motor impairments. Emergency neuroimaging should be performed on all patients with a postictal focal deficit or change in mental status that does not quickly resolve.

When Should Treatment Be Started?

If the diagnosis of epilepsy cannot be established, one should obtain further testing and diagnostic information. One option is to obtain additional EEG recordings, although often one must simply wait and observe a patient over an extended period of time before reaching a diagnosis. Once epilepsy has been diagnosed, an antiepileptic drug (AED) appropriate for that condition may be prescribed. If only one seizure has occurred, then the decision to treat rests on both the probability of recurrence and type of seizure experienced. Patients who are at significant risk for recurrence are usually offered treatment, whereas patients who have a low probability of recurrence may not be started on medication. The seizure type also influences the decision. Tonic-clonic seizures or other seizure types that cause loss of consciousness or falling are intrinsically more dangerous than seizures without those characteristics. For example, a patient who experiences a tonic-clonic seizure is far more likely to fear the consequences of another seizure than a patient whose seizure consisted of tingling or twitching of a hand for several seconds. Therefore, the decision to treat must be made by the physician in consultation with the patient, because the latter is the one who will suffer the risks of seizures, the side effects of medication, and the psychosocial consequences of additional seizures. Children usually live in a somewhat sheltered environment; a second seizure therefore has different consequences for a child than for most adults, who must function independently and have weightier responsibilities. Therefore, physicians often advise waiting until a second seizure has occurred when seeing a child after a first seizure unless the probability of recurrence is high. In contrast, adults more often desire treatment to minimize the risk of recurrence, thereby maximizing their chances of continued full function in society.

A patient who has had a *single* seizure, with a normal developmental history, neurological examination, EEG, neuroimaging study, and no family history of epilepsy, is often simply observed and medication is not prescribed. The risk of a recurrent seizure after a single seizure in this circumstance is approximately 25%–30% (Figure 1.1). After one seizure with an abnormal EEG or evidence of some other neurological abnormality, the risk for recurrence may be 50% or greater. After two seizures, the risk of recurrent seizures increases to 75%–85%, and treatment is often advised after a second seizure has occurred and may be started after one seizure if an individual has a heightened risk for recurrence. Predictors of recurrence after the first seizure are summarized in Box 1.2. If more than one seizure has occurred, then the probability of recurrence is quite high, and treatment is usually offered,

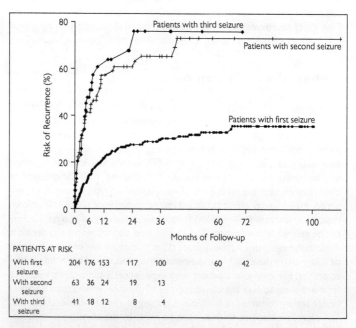

Figure 1.1 Risk of a second, third, and fourth unprovoked seizure after a first, second, and third unprovoked seizure. Reprinted with permission (Hauser, Rich, Lee, Annegers, & Anderson, 1998).

> **Box 1.2 Predictors of Increased Risk for Recurrence After the First Seizure**
>
> - Prior neurological insult (mental retardation, cerebral palsy): the most powerful predictor of recurrence
> - Partial-onset (focal) seizures
> - Abnormal electroencephalogram
> - Prior acute seizures including febrile seizures
> - Status epilepticus or multiple seizures at the index episode (in adults)
> - Postictal Todd's paralysis
>
> From Chadwick (2006), Hauser (2006), and Shorvon and Luciano (2007).

although this also depends on seizure type, because some seizures might be so mild and inconsequential as to merit simple observation without treatment.

Selection and Adjustment of Medication

The goal of treatment is to prevent future seizures from recurring. Treatment is typically started with one of the first-line AEDs (see Chapters 2 and 5). First-line drugs should be effective and well tolerated. For localization-related epilepsy (partial onset seizures), these drugs include carbamazepine, lacosamide, lamotrigine, levetiracetam, oxcarbazepine, and phenytoin, among others. For generalized epilepsies, first-line drugs include ethosuximide, lamotrigine, levetiracetam, topiramate, and valproate, among others. If a first-line drug controls seizures and does not cause side effects, therapeutic adjustments are not needed. Should seizures persist, the medication regimen should be adjusted (see Chapter 8). If a patient has significant side effects, then the physician should advise switching to an alternative AED. One should aim for treatment with a single agent (monotherapy), to lessen the chances of adverse effects and drug interactions.

A therapeutic range of serum concentration exists for all drugs. This range, in theory, provides a guideline for determining the appropriate dose. Serum levels below certain concentrations are undoubtedly ineffective. Excessively high serum levels will certainly produce unwanted side effects. However, the therapeutic range may differ from one patient to the next, and the lower limits are not well established for any drug. It is critical that patients be treated based on symptoms—prevention of seizures and lack of side effects—and not the plasma drug level (see Chapter 4).

Other Treatment Possibilities

Approximately 35% of individuals with epilepsy have persistent seizures despite the use of appropriate AEDs. Once adequate trials of two tolerated, appropriately chosen and used AED schedules (whether as monotherapies or in combination) have failed to achieve sustained seizure freedom, other treatment options should be considered (Kwan et al., 2010). First, diagnostic testing should be performed to verify the diagnosis of epilepsy and to ensure that the patient does not have psychogenic non-epileptic seizures or some other disorder. If drug-resistant epilepsy is confirmed, then several treatment options exist. Epilepsy surgery is the only treatment that offers a good chance of stopping seizures completely, and the other options are palliative. *Epilepsy surgery* usually involves either excising the cortical area that causes seizures or disconnecting epileptogenic regions of the brain from other areas. Removal of part of the temporal lobe, anterior temporal lobectomy, or anterome-dial temporal resection are the operations most commonly performed, but surgery can often be carried out in other lobes of the brain as well. Disconnection procedures, such as a corpus callosotomy, also can be done. This is generally palliative and works best for refractory tonic, atonic, and tonic-clonic seizures. Other treatment options include *vagal nerve stimulation*, a mainly palliative treatment that electrically stimulates the left vagus nerve in the neck. The ketogenic diet is a diet that excludes carbohydrates and consists of foods with a fat-to-protein ratio of 3.5:1 or 4:1, so that the body metabo-lizes ketones instead of glucose. This may lessen seizure frequency in about half of the people who use it and occasionally stops seizures completely; it is mainly used in children but can be prescribed for motivated adults. New treatments are being studied and developed using electrical stimulation of various areas of the brain to suppress seizures.

Discontinuing Antiepileptic Drug Therapy

Once a patient has been free of seizures for an extended period of time, withdrawal of medication may be considered. However, risk of recurrence of seizures should be discussed with the patient (Figure 1.2). The decision to stop medication must be individualized and is based on the epilepsy

Figure 1.2 Actuarial percentage of seizure-free patients stopping treatment or con-tinuing treatment. Reprinted with permission (Specchio et al., 2002).

> ### Box 1.3 Predictors of Increased Risk for Relapse After Drug Withdrawal
>
> - Older age at onset: onset as an adolescent or adult
> - Seizures after initiation of treatment
> - Long interval between onset and initial control
> - Many generalized seizures before control
> - Partial or secondary generalized seizures
> - Myoclonic seizures
> - Need for multiple antiepileptic drugs (AEDs)
> - Short duration of remission before medication taper
> - Abnormal neurological examination (cerebral palsy, mental retardation)
> - Known cause for epilepsy
> - Abnormal electroencephalogram (EEG) at diagnosis, particularly a spike-wave pattern
> - Presence of abnormal EEG after starting treatment
> - Worsening of EEG findings during medication taper
>
> From Chadwick (2006), Hauser (2006), and Shorvon and Luciano (2007).

syndrome and probability of seizure recurrence (Box 1.3), the associated risks (both medical and psychosocial) of seizure recurrence, and the risks of continuing medical therapy. It is typical to require a minimum of 2 years without seizures before considering discontinuation of medical therapy, although some physicians prefer to wait longer. Medication dosages are usually gradually reduced and withdrawn over a period of at least 6 weeks, but longer periods are often advised. Rapid withdrawal of some medications, particularly the barbiturates, is potentially dangerous, because this can precipitate seizures (see Chapter 2).

When to Seek Specialist Consultation

Neurology consultation is useful when the diagnosis is uncertain or if one AED has failed to completely control seizures. Other indications for consultation include family planning or if the patient has a form of epilepsy that is particularly difficult to treat. An epilepsy specialist should be consulted if two AEDs fail to control seizures or the diagnosis remains in doubt.

References

Asadi-Pooya AA, Nikseresht AR, Yaghoobi E. Vasovagal syncope treated as epilepsy for 16 years. *Iran J Med Sci*, 2011; 36(1): 60–62.

Asadi-Pooya AA, Emami M. Reasons for uncontrolled seizures in children; the impact of pseudointractability. *Epilepsy Behav*, 2012; 25(3): 341–344.

Asadi-Pooya AA, Emami M, Sperling MR. A clinical study of syndromes of idiopathic (genetic) generalized epilepsy. *J Neurol Sci*, 2013; 324(1-2): 113–117.

Asadi-Pooya AA, Emami M, Ashjazadeh N, Nikseresht A, Shariat A, Petramfar P, Yousefipour G, Borhani-Haghighi A, Izadi S, Rahimi-Jaberi A. Reasons for uncontrolled seizures in adults; the impact of pseudointractability. *Seizure*, 2013; 22(4): 271–274

Berg AT, Berkovic SF, Brodie MJ, et al. Revised terminology and concepts for organization of seizures and epilepsies: Report of the ILAE Commission on Classification and Terminology, 2005–2009. *Epilepsia*, 2010; 51:676–685.

Blume WT, Luders H, Mizrahi E, Tassinari C, van Emde Boas W, Engel J. Glossary of descriptive terminology for ictal semiology: report of the ILAE Task Force on Classification and Terminology. *Epilepsia*, 2001;42:1212–1218.

Chadwick D. Starting and stopping treatment for seizures and epilepsy. *Epilepsia*, 2006;47(Suppl 1):58–61.

Engel J. ILAE Classification of epilepsy syndromes. *Epilepsy Research*, 2006; 70S:S5–S10.

Fisher RS, Acevedo C, Arzimanoglou A, Bogacz A, Cross JH, Elger CE, Engel J Jr, Forsgren L, French JA, Glynn M, Hesdorffer DC, Lee BI, Mathern GW, Moshé SL, Perucca E, Scheffer IE, Tomson T, Watanabe M, Wiebe S. ILAE official report: a practical clinical definition of epilepsy. *Epilepsia*, 2014;55(4):475–482.

Hauser WA. The natural history of seizures. In Wyllie E, ed. *The Treatment of Epilepsy: Principles and Practice* (pp 117–124), 4th ed. Lippincott Williams & Wilkins, Philadelphia, 2006.

Hauser WA, Rich SS, Lee JRJ, Annegers JF, Anderson VE. Risk of recurrent seizures after two unprovoked seizures. *New England Journal of Medicine*, 1998;338:429–434.

International League Against Epilepsy: *A proposed diagnostic schema for people with epileptic seizures and with epilepsy: Report of the ILAE Task Force on Classification and Terminology*. Retrieved from http://www.ilae-epilepsy.org/Visitors/Centre/ctf/.

Kwan P, Arzimanoglou A, Berg AT, Brodie MJ, et al. Definition of drug resistant epilepsy: consensus proposal by the ad hoc Task Force of the ILAE Commission on Therapeutic Strategies. *Epilepsia*, 2010; 51 (6): 1069–1077.

Shorvon S, Luciano AL. Prognosis of chronic and newly diagnosed epilepsy: revisiting temporal aspects. *Current Opinions in Neurology*, 2007;20:208–212.

Specchio LM, Tramacere L, LaNeve A, Beghi E. Discontinuing antiepileptic drugs in patients who are seizure free on monotherapy. *Journal of Neurology, Neurosurgery, and Psychiatry*, 2002;72:22–25.

Chapter 2

Antiepileptic Drug Dosage Forms and Administration Guidelines

In this chapter, dosage forms, starting dose, titration schedule, maintenance dose, dose limits, and discontinuation schedule of each antiepileptic drug (AED) are discussed separately. In addition, significant administration guidelines, contraindications, precautions, and information for patients are discussed briefly. Indications for each of AEDs are discussed in Chapter 5.

Key Points for Prescribing Antiepileptic Drugs

- Choose an AED that is appropriate for the seizure type and epilepsy syndrome. Because there often are several good options, choose the specific agent based on the patient's profile (i.e., gender, age, job, etc.), comorbidity, potential side effects, drug interactions, and other pharmacological properties.
- When beginning therapy with an AED, first target the lower end of the therapeutic range or dose. Use higher doses only when lower ones have failed. This approach lessens the incidence of side effects.
- Titrate doses gradually when initiating therapy to improve drug tolerability and reduce side effects. Controlled studies show evidence of efficacy during drug titration, even though full therapeutic levels may not yet be achieved.
- If needed for immediate seizure control, levetiracetam, oxcarbazepine, phenytoin, rufinamide, topiramate, valproate, and zonisamide can be rapidly titrated.
- Tailor dosing schedules to provide maximum protection (peak levels) when seizures are apt to occur. For example, if seizures typically occur in the morning after awakening (as in juvenile myoclonic epilepsy), dose the medication at bedtime so that maximal levels are present on awakening. If divided doses are used, prescribe the larger amount shortly before seizures are likely to occur (ie, at the time of greatest vulnerability).

- If dividing a daily dose leads to unequal amounts at different dosing times, prescribe the larger dose either shortly before seizures are most likely to occur or at bedtime; bedtime dosing is often preferred when seizures occur randomly at any time, because peak concentration side effects are less likely to be noticed when asleep. For example, if phenytoin 300 mg is the total daily dose, prescribe 100 mg to be taken in the morning and 200 mg to be taken at night.
- It is preferable to prescribe medications that can be taken once or twice daily. Patient adherence to a medication regimen is highest with once- or twice-daily dosing regimens.
- Observe closely for side effects. Development of adverse effects is a common reason for poor adherence (compliance) to a prescribed regimen. Because patients are often unaware of cognitive or behavioral side effects, question family members and close friends about side effects as well.
- The goal of treatment is to prevent seizures and avoid side effects. Assess whether these goals have been met. If not, adjust therapy accordingly. If the first drug fails, convert the patient to monotherapy on a new agent. If a second drug fails, either convert to mono-therapy with a new agent or consider adding a second drug to the existing agent. (There are no data to support superiority of one course of action over another.)
- When converting from monotherapy from one drug to another, the following procedure can be used: Titrate the new AED to a therapeutic dose, lowering the dose of the first drug modestly (10%–25%) to avoid side effects. One should maintain reasonably therapeutic levels of the original AED while titrating the new agent to avoid seizure exacerbation. Should side effects appear during titration of the new agent, first try and reduce the dose of the original drug, since many side effects are likely due to transient polypharmacy rather than an effect of the new drug. Should side effects persist, however, they may be caused by the new agent, and this may need to be discontinued. Once the new AED is at a therapeutic dose or level without significant untoward side effects, then taper the original drug over 6 weeks or so (longer if a barbiturate or benzodiazepine).
- Once two appropriate drugs prescribed either singly or in combination have failed, consider epilepsy surgery after confirming the diagnosis of epilepsy.
- If epilepsy surgery cannot be performed, consider alternative therapies such as trials of other AEDs, vagus nerve stimulation, ketogenic diet, or investigational therapies.

Acetazolamide

Brand Name: Diamox®.

Dosage Forms: Tablets 125 mg, 250 mg (Tablet is no longer available in the USA).

Note: The extended-release preparation is not recommended for use as an AED.

Dosage

Starting Dose
Adults and children: 4–8 mg/kg/day, given in two divided doses. When given in combination with other AEDs, the recommended starting dosage in adults is 250 mg twice daily. *Elderly:* Consider dosage reduction.

Maintenance Dose: The usual maintenance dose is 375–1500 mg/day or 8–30 mg/kg/day. An elderly patient, with an age-related renal impairment, is more likely to develop hyperchloremic metabolic acidosis; therefore, use lower doses.

Maximum Dosage Limit: *In all age groups:* 1500 mg/day.

Discontinuation Schedule: A dosage reduction of 50% per two weeks is safe at the time of discontinuation.

Administration Guidelines
May be taken with or without food. To prepare an oral liquid for patients who are unable to take tablets, crush tablets and suspend in any highly flavored carbohydrate syrup (e.g., cherry or chocolate). Up to 500 mg may be suspended in 5 mL of syrup; however, concentrations of 250 mg/5 mL are more palatable. The resultant suspensions are stable for about 1 week.

Patient Education

1. If you miss a dose, take it as soon as you can. If it is almost time for your next dose, take only that dose. Do not take double or extra doses.
2. Side effects that you should report to your physician as soon as possible include

    blood in urine, pain or difficulty passing urine

    black tarry stools

    dark yellow or brown urine, pale stools, yellowing of the eyes or skin

    confusion or depression

    difficulty breathing, shortness of breath

    dry mouth or increased thirst

    fatigue or severe lack of energy

    fever, sore throat

    lower back pain

    muscle weakness

    ringing in the ears

    seizures

    skin rash, itching

    unusual bleeding or bruising

    irregular heart beat.

3. Do not stop taking acetazolamide suddenly. Your physician may want you to reduce your dose gradually.
4. You may get drowsy. Do not drive, use machinery, or do anything that needs mental alertness, until you know how acetazolamide affects you.

5. Drink several glasses of water a day. This will help to reduce possible kidney problems.
6. If you are diabetic, monitor blood and urine sugar and ketones regularly. Acetazolamide can increase sugar levels. Report to your physician if you notice any changes.

See Box 2.1 and Box 2.2.

Box 2.1 Relative Contraindications to Use of Acetazolamide

- Adrenal insufficiency
- Renal diseases
- Anuria
- Renal failure
- Marked hepatic disease
- Hyperchloremic metabolic acidosis
- Electrolyte imbalances
    - Hypokalemia
    - Hyponatremia
- Acetazolamide hypersensitivity

See Chapters 12, 13, and 14.

Box 2.2 Acetazolamide Precautions

- Breastfeeding
- Pregnancy
- Elderly
- Pulmonary diseases
- Hematological diseases
- Sulfonamide hypersensitivity
- Sunlight or ultraviolet exposure

See Chapters 9, 10, 11, 18, and 26.

For the explanation of the contraindications and precautions of each drug, please go to the appropriate chapter. For example, for the explanation of *marked hepatic disease* as a relative contraindication for prescribing *acetazolamide*, see Chapter 13.

Benzodiazepines

Clonazepam
Brand Names: Klonopin®.

Dosage Forms: Tablets 0.5 mg, 1 mg, 2 mg; Wafers (orally disintegrating tablets) 0.125 mg, 0.25 mg, 0.5 mg, 1 mg, 2 mg.

Dosage

Starting Dose

Adults and adolescents (weight ≥30 kg or 10 years of age or older): 0.5–1.0 mg/ day, divided in two equal doses or just at bedtime.

Elderly and debilitated adult patients: May require lower initial dosages.

Children and infants (weight <30 kg or up to 10 years of age): 0.01–0.03 mg/ kg/day (not to exceed 0.05 mg/kg/day), given orally in two or three equally divided doses.

Titration and Maintenance Dose: In adults and adolescents, dosage may be increased by 0.5–1 mg every 3–7 days until seizures are controlled or adverse reactions limit further increase. The typical maintenance dose range is 2–8 mg/day. In elderly and debilitated adult patients slower dosage titration is recommended. In children and infants, increase dosage by not more than 0.25–0.5 mg every 3 days to a maximum maintenance dosage of 0.1–0.2 mg/kg/day administered in 2 or 3 divided doses until seizures are controlled or adverse reactions limit further increase. Sometimes, bedtime dosing alone is sufficient.

Maximum Dosage Limits

- *Adults and adolescents (weight ≥30 kg):* 20 mg/day.
- *Children and infants (weight <30 kg):* 0.2 mg/kg/day.

Discontinuation Schedule: A dosage reduction of 0.04 mg/kg per month is safe at the time of discontinuation.

Administration Guidelines

Clonazepam may be administered orally without regard to meals.
Conventional oral tablets: Should be swallowed whole with a glass of water.

Disintegrating tablet: Make sure hands are dry before touching the tablet. Peel foil back from blister package. Do not push tablet through the foil. Place tablet in mouth and tablet should melt quickly. You may drink some water after tablet melts.

Patient Education

1. If you miss a dose and remember within an hour, take it as soon as you can. If it is more than an hour since you missed a dose, skip that dose and go back to your regular schedule. Do not take double or extra doses.
2. Side effects that you should report to your physician as soon as possible include

   confusion or drowsiness

   unusual behavior or thoughts of hurting yourself

   worsening seizures

   double vision or abnormal eye movements

   hallucinations (seeing and hearing things that are not really there)

   lightheadedness or fainting spells

    mood changes, depression, excitability, or aggressive behavior

    movement difficulty, staggering or jerky movements

    muscle cramps

    restlessness

    tremors

    weakness or tiredness.

3. Your body may become dependent on clonazepam. If you have been taking clonazepam regularly for some time, do not suddenly stop taking it. You must gradually reduce the dose or you may get severe adverse effects.

4. You may get drowsy or dizzy. Do not drive, use machinery, or do anything that needs mental alertness until you know how clonazepam affects you. To reduce the risk of dizzy and fainting spells, do not sit or stand up quickly. Alcohol may increase dizziness and drowsiness. Avoid alcoholic drinks.

5. Do not treat yourself for coughs, colds, or allergies without asking your physician for advice. Some ingredients can increase possible adverse effects.

6. If you are going to have surgery, tell your physician that you are taking clonazepam.

See Box 2.3 and Box 2.4.

Box 2.3 Relative Contraindications to Use of Clonazepam

- Abrupt discontinuation
- Benzodiazepine hypersensitivity
- Ethanol intoxication
- Acute respiratory insufficiency

Box 2.4 Clonazepam Precautions

- Bipolar disorder
- Depression
- Psychosis
- Suicidal ideation
- Benzodiazepine dependence
- Substance abuse
- Elderly
- Pregnancy
- Obstetric delivery
- Breastfeeding

- Central nervous system depression and coma
- Dementia
- Chronic pulmonary diseases
- Sleep apnea
- Neuromuscular diseases (e.g., myasthenia gravis)
- Parkinson's disease
- Hepatic diseases
- Renal impairment
- Shock

See Chapters 9–13, 22, and 23.

Diazepam

Brand Names: Diastat® AcuDial™, Valium®, Diazepam Intensol.™

Dosage Forms: Tablets 2 mg, 5 mg, 10 mg; Solution 1 mg/mL, 5 mg/mL; Injection 5 mg/mL; Rectal gel Diastat® 5 mg/ml, Diastat® AcuDial™ 10 mg (delivers set doses of 5 mg, 7.5 mg, and 10 mg), Diastat® AcuDial™ 20 mg (delivers set doses of 10 mg, 12.5 mg, 15 mg, 17.5 mg, and 20 mg).

Dosage

Intravenous (IV) dosage for the treatment of status epilepticus
Adults and adolescents: 10–20 mg IV over 2–5 minutes; may be repeated at 10–15 minute intervals (usually for two doses), to a maximum dosage of 30 mg.

Children >5 years: 0.1–0.3 mg/kg IV over 3–5 minutes; could be given every 10–15 minutes (usually for two doses), to a maximum total dose of 15 mg. *Children and infants 1 month–5 years:* 0.1–0.3 mg/kg IV over 3–5 minutes; could be repeated every 2–5 minutes (usually for two doses), to a maximum dose of 5 mg.

Neonates: 0.1–0.3 mg/kg IV over 3–5 minutes; could be given every 15–30 minutes (usually for two doses), to a maximum total dose of 2 mg.

Note: Not recommended as a first-line agent in neonates due to sodium benzoate and benzoic acid in the injection.

Note: Many clinicians now prefer IV lorazepam to IV diazepam for the acute treatment of seizures.

Oral (PO) dosage for adjunctive treatment of seizures and intermittent (in cycles lasting 3 weeks) use of diazepam to control clusters or bouts of increased seizure activity in refractory partial or generalized epilepsies.
Children and infants ≥ 6 months: 1–2.5 mg PO 3–4 times per day (0.5–0.75 mg/kg/day). The dose may be increased as needed and tolerated.

Adults and adolescents: 2–10 mg PO 2–4 times per day only during a seizure cluster. In general, we prefer using lorazepam for seizure clusters if an oral preparation can be taken rather than diazepam. We advise against using diazepam as adjunctive therapy, and prefer it only for treating seizure clusters.

Elderly: 2–2.5 mg PO 1–2 times per day for seizure clusters. Increase the dose according to response and patient tolerability.

Note: For febrile seizure prophylaxis in children and infants 6 months–5 years, oral diazepam 0.33 mg/kg is given every 8 hours (1 mg/kg/day) during each episode of fever until the child is afebrile for at least 24 hours.

Rectal (PR) dosage in acute repetitive seizures
Children 2–5 years: 0.5 mg/kg PR. Doses should be rounded upward to the next available dosage strength. If needed, a second dose may be given 4–12 hours after the first dose.

Children 6–11 years: 0.3 mg/kg PR. Doses should be rounded upward to the next available dosage strength. If needed, a second dose may be given 4–12 hours after the first dose.

Adults and adolescents: 0.2 mg/kg (usually 10–20 mg) PR. Doses should be rounded upward to the next available dosage strength. If needed, a second dose may be given 4–12 hours after the first dose.

Elderly and debilitated patients: 0.2 mg/kg PR. Doses should be rounded downward to reduce the adverse effects. If needed, a second dose may be given 4–12 hours after the first dose.

Note: It is recommended that rectal diazepam be used to treat no more than five episodes per month and no more than one episode every 5 days.

Note: A 2.5-mg dose may also be used as a partial replacement dose for patients who expel a portion of the first dose.

Maximum Dosage Limits: This must be individualized, generally not more than 20 mg as a single dose.

Administration Guidelines

Following parenteral administration, patient should be kept under close observation for a period of 3–8 hours or longer, based on the patient's clinical response and rate of recovery.

> Replace parenteral therapy with oral therapy as soon as possible.
> *Intramuscular injection* is not recommended due to slow and erratic absorption.

For *intravenous injection,* do not administer rapidly because respiratory depression or hypotension may develop. In adults, inject IV slowly at a rate not exceeding 5 mg/min. In Infants and children, inject IV at a rate not exceeding 1–2 mg/min. Monitor heart rate, respiratory rate, and blood pressure. A large vein should be used to avoid thrombosis. If a large vein is not available, inject into the tubing of a flowing IV solution as close as possible to the vein insertion. Do not add diazepam emulsified injection to infusion sets containing PVC.

Lorazepam

Brand Names: Ativan®, Lorazepam Intensol™.

Dosage Forms: Tablets 0.5 mg, 1 mg, 2 mg; Injection 2 mg/mL, 4 mg/mL; Oral Solution (Lorazepam Intensol™) 2 mg/mL.

Dosage

Dosage for the treatment of status epilepticus
Adults: 0.1 mg/kg IV given at a rate of approximately 2 mg per minute, ceasing infusion when seizures stop. A second dose of 0.05 mg/kg may be given after 10–15 minutes if needed. If this is ineffective, additional doses may be given, but we generally advise adding a second agent after failure of 0.15 mg/kg of intravenous lorazepam.

Adolescents: 0.07 mg/kg IV given slowly over 2–5 minutes (no more than 2 mg/min). A second dose of 0.05 mg/kg may be given after 10–15 minutes if needed. *Children and infants:* 0.1 mg/kg (maximum 4 mg) IV given slowly over 2–5 minutes. A second dose of 0.05 mg/kg IV may be repeated after 10–15 minutes if needed. *Neonates:* 0.05 mg/kg IV slowly over 2–5 minutes. Second dose may be given after 10–15 minutes if needed.

Note: Intramuscular administration is not a preferred route for status epilepticus since therapeutic levels may not be reached as quickly as intravenous administration. However, if the intravenous route is unavailable, then the intramuscular route can be utilized. Lorazepam injection, undiluted, should be injected deep into the muscle mass when given intramuscularly. However, rectal diazepam is probably preferred if an intravenous route is not available.

Note: Lorazepam injection contains benzyl alcohol, which may be toxic to neonates in high doses.

Oral (PO) dosage for adjunctive treatment of seizures and intermittent (in cycles lasting 3 weeks) use of lorazepam to control clusters or bouts of increased seizure activity in refractory partial or generalized epilepsies

Adults and adolescents: 1–3 mg PO 1–2 times per day only during a seizure cluster. In general, we prefer using lorazepam for seizure clusters if an oral preparation can be taken rather than diazepam, because of its longer duration of anticonvulsant action in the central nervous system.

Administration Guidelines

Do not administer lorazepam injection by intra-arterial injection because arteriospasm can occur, which may cause tissue damage.

Rate of injection should not exceed 2 mg/min. Dilute IV dose with equal volume of compatible diluents (D5W, NS, SWI). Direct IV injection should be made with repeated aspiration to ensure that none of the drug is injected intra-arterially and that perivascular extravasation does not occur.

For *continuous IV infusion,* when PVC containers or administration sets are used to administer lorazepam, significant drug losses occur due to sorption. Use of glass or polyolefin containers is recommended.

Midazolam

Brand Name: Versed®.

Dosage Forms: Injection 1 mg/mL, 5 mg/mL; syrup 2 mg/mL.

Dosage

Dosage for the treatment of refractory status epilepticus:
Adults (for mechanically ventilated patients only): 0.2 mg/kg IV bolus followed by a continuous infusion of 0.75 µg/kg/min IV. Dose should be

titrated upward every 5 minutes until seizures are controlled (up to 10 µg/kg/min IV). The infusion is maintained for 12 hours and slowly tapered during continuous EEG monitoring. If seizure activity returns, the infusion is restarted for another 12 hours. Tolerance may develop and doses up to 20 µg/kg/min IV are sometimes required.

Children and infants >2 months (for mechanically ventilated patients only): 0.15 mg/kg (0.1–0.3 mg/kg) IV bolus followed by a continuous infusion of 1 µg/kg/min IV. Dose should be titrated upward every 5 minutes until seizures are controlled (up to 5 µg/kg/min IV). The infusion is maintained for 12 hours and slowly tapered during continuous EEG monitoring. If seizure activity returns, the infusion is restarted for another 12 hours. Occasionally, several days of high-dose (up to 20 µg/kg/min IV) therapy is required. In neonates, doses of 0.1–0.4 mg/kg/hour are used in patients refractory to high doses of phenobarbital.

Administration Guidelines

Intramuscular, intranasal, and buccal midazolam (10 mg in adults and 0.2 mg/kg in children) routes are useful in acute repetitive seizures and febrile seizures in children. For buccal route, dilute 10 mg midazolam with peppermint, swirl in the mouth for 4–5 minutes, and then spit out.

Nitrazepam

Dosage Forms: Tablet 5 mg, oral suspension 2.5 mg/5ml.

This drug is often used in children (myoclonic seizures from West syndrome, Lennox-Gastaut syndrome).

Dosage:

Starting Dose:

   Children and infants (weight < 30 kg): 0.25 mg/kg/day in 2-3 divided doses.

Titration and maintenance dose:
In children and infants increase dosage 0.25 mg / kg / day every 2 weeks, until seizures are controlled or adverse reactions limit further increase.

Maximum Dosage Limits:
Children and infants (weight < 30 kg): 3 mg/kg/day.

Discontinuation schedule: As with all benzodiazepines, abrupt withdrawal may precipitate seizures.

Note: In case of prolonged therapy, for all benzodiazepines a dosage reduction of 20%–25% per month is safe at the time of discontinuation.

Clobazam

Brand Name: Frisium®, Onfi®.

Dosage Forms: Tablets 10 mg and 20 mg; Oral Suspension: 2.5 mg/mL.

Dosage:

Starting Dose:

Adults and adolescents: 5–10 mg/day, in 1–2 doses.
Elderly and debilitated adult patients: Lower initial doses.
Children and infants (weight < 30 kg): 0.25 mg/kg/day in 2 divided doses.

Titration and maintenance dose:
In adults and adolescents dosage may be increased by 5–15 mg every 5 days until seizures are controlled or adverse reactions limit further increase. The typical maintenance dose ranges 20–40 mg/day. In elderly and debilitated adult patients slower dosage titration is recommended. In children and infants increase dosage gradually every 5 days, until seizures are controlled or adverse reactions limit further increase.

Maximum Dosage Limits:

- Adults and adolescents (weight > 30 kg): 80 mg/day.
- Children and infants (weight < 30 kg): 1 mg/kg/day.

Discontinuation schedule: As with all benzodiazepines, abrupt withdrawal may precipitate seizures.

Note: In case of prolonged therapy, for all benzodiazepines a dosage reduction of 20%–25% per month is safe at the time of discontinuation.

Carbamazepine

Brand Names: Carbatrol®, Epitol®, Equetro®, Tegretol®, Tegretol®-XR.

Dosage Forms

Carbamazepine (Tegretol®): Tablets 200 mg; Chewable tablets 100 mg; Oral suspension 100 mg/5 mL.

Epitol®: Tablet 200 mg.

Tegretol®-XR: Tablets 100 mg, 200 mg, 400 mg.

Carbatrol®: Capsule-XR 100 mg, 200 mg, 300 mg.

Dosage

Starting Dose
Adults and adolescents: 100–200 mg twice daily.

Children 6–12 years: 100 mg twice daily (or 50 mg four times per day of suspension) or 10 mg/kg/day given in 2 divided doses for tablets, or 4 divided doses for the suspension.

Children <6 years: 10 mg/kg/day divided in 2 or 3 daily doses for tablets, or 4 divided doses for the suspension.

Titration and Maintenance Dose

Adults and adolescents: Increase 200 mg/day every 5–7 days; give daily dose in 2 divided doses for extended release preparation and 2–4 divided doses for the regular preparation. Effective range is generally 400–1200 mg/day (7–15 mg/kg/day), though higher doses can be used if serum levels remain low.

Children 6–12 years: Increase by 100 mg/day at 5–7 day intervals; give daily dose in 2 divided doses for the extended release preparation and 2–4 divided doses for the regular preparation. Dose should be adjusted to the minimum effective level. The usual maintenance dosage range is 15–30 mg/kg/day.

Children <6 years: Increase weekly as needed; most patients will respond to doses below 35 mg/kg/day. If satisfactory response is not achieved, plasma drug concentrations should be checked to ensure adequate plasma levels. The safety of doses above 35–40 mg/kg/day has not been established.

Note: Extended-release tablets (Tegretol®-XR) are not recommended in children below 6 years of age by manufacturers, but this is because testing has not been done and it may be difficult for young children to swallow a tablet rather than use the chewable 100-mg pill or the suspension. Children less than 12 years old who receive greater than or equal to 400 mg/day of carbamazepine may be converted to extended release formulations using the same total daily dosage divided twice daily.

Note: Periodic monitoring of serum carbamazepine concentrations is recommended.

Note: A loading dose is not generally recommended.

Maximum Dosage Limits: These are dependent on serum level, and because of autoinduction of hepatic microsomal enzymes, dosage guidelines vary from one patient to the next.

- *Adults and elderly:* 1600 mg/day (higher doses can be used depending on serum levels).
- *Adolescents >15 years:* 1200 mg/day (higher doses can be used depending on serum levels).
- *Children and adolescents 6–15 years:* 1000 mg/day (depending on serum level).
- *Children <6 years:* 35–40 mg/kg/day.

Discontinuation Schedule: A dosage reduction of 20%–25% per 1–2 weeks is a safe discontinuation regimen.

Administration Guidelines

Administer with meals or with a large amount of water to minimize gastrointestinal side effects. May need to split doses to avoid GI upset.

For administration of suspension via nasogastric or enteral feeding tubes: To minimize any interaction that might occur with enteral feedings, turn off feedings at least 15 minutes before and hold for 15 minutes after a dose. Flush the tube with 15–30 mL (in adults) of water, D_5W, or NS prior to administration. To minimize the loss of drug, dilute the suspension with an equal volume of water prior to administration. Follow dose administration with flushing the tube with an additional 15–30 mL (in adults) of water, D_5W, or NS. Do not administer carbamazepine suspension with any other liquid medications or diluents since combination with other suspensions may form precipitants with loss of bioavailability.

For conversion from oral tablets/capsules to oral suspension: Patients should be converted to the suspension from the oral tablets or capsules by administering the same number of mg per day in smaller, more frequent doses (e.g., changing from twice per day for tablets to four times per day for the suspension).

Patient Education

1. If you miss a dose, take it as soon as you can. If it is almost time for your next dose, take only that dose. Do not take double or extra doses.
2. Side effects that you should report to your physician as soon as possible include:
   blurred or double vision, uncontrollable eye movements
   chest pain or tightness
   difficulty breathing or shortness of breath, wheezing
   fainting spells
   fast or irregular heartbeat (palpitations)
   dark yellow or brown urine
   pain or difficulty passing urine
   increased thirst
   mouth ulcers
   fever or chills, sore throat
   redness, blistering, peeling or loosening of the skin, including inside the mouth
   skin rash, hives, itching
   seizures
   stomach pain
   vomiting
   yellowing of the eyes or skin
   swollen joints or muscle/joint aches and pains
   unusual bleeding or bruising
   ringing in the ears
   confusion
   lightheadedness
   mood changes, nervousness, or hostility
   unusual tiredness or weakness.

3. Do not change brands or dosage forms of carbamazepine without discussing the change with your physician.

4. You may get drowsy, dizzy, or have blurred vision. Do not drive, use machinery, or do anything that needs mental alertness until you know how carbamazepine affects you. To reduce dizzy or fainting spells, do not sit or stand up quickly. Alcohol can increase drowsiness and dizziness. Avoid alcoholic drinks.

5. If you are female and are taking birth control pills or other hormonal birth control methods (like injections), you should know that the birth control might not work as well while you are taking carbamazepine. Discuss this issue with your physician.

6. Carbamazepine may make your skin more sensitive to the sun or ultraviolet light. Keep out of the sun, or wear protective clothing outdoors and use a sunscreen (at least SPF 15). Do not use sun lamps or sun tanning beds or booths.

7. If you are going to have surgery, tell your physician that you are taking carbamazepine.

See Box 2.5 and Box 2.6.

Box 2.5 Relative Contraindications to Use of Carbamazepine

- Bone marrow suppression
- Atrioventricular block or bundle-branch block
- Carbamazepine hypersensitivity
- Tricyclic antidepressant hypersensitivity
- Monoamine oxidase inhibitor therapy

See Chapters 17 and 18.

Box 2.6 Carbamazepine Precautions

- Atonic seizures
- Absence seizure
- Myoclonic seizures
- Barbiturate hypersensitivity
- Hydantoin hypersensitivity
- Breastfeeding
- Pregnancy
- Neonates
- Elderly
- Abrupt discontinuation
- Psychosis
- Alcoholism
- Glaucoma and increased intra-ocular pressure
- Hepatic diseases
- Hypercholesterolemia
- Hyponatremia
- Artery diseases
- Renal diseases
- Sunlight or ultraviolet exposure

See Chapters 7, 9–15, 17, 18, and 26.

Corticotropin, ACTH

Brand Names: Acthar®, H.P. Acthar®.

Dosage Forms: Repository corticotrophin injection: 80 units/mL (in 5-mL multidose vials).

Dosage

Infants with infantile spasm: Various regimens have been used. Low-doses of 5–40 units/day IM for 1–6 weeks have been recommended by some neurologists, while others recommend larger doses of 40–160 units/day IM for 3–12 months. The usual dosage range is 20–40 units/day (50–100 IU/m^2) IM or 5–8 units/kg/day IM in two divided doses for 1–3 weeks. If response is complete, taper ACTH over 1–4 months. If response is observed but is incomplete increase the dose to 60–80 IU/day (150–200 IU/m^2) for 2 weeks. If spasms and hypsarrhythmia resolve, ACTH should be tapered over 1–4 months. If relapse occurs during tapering, the dose may be increased to the previously effective dose for 2 weeks and then another tapering begun. If therapy at these doses is not successful, ACTH should be rapidly tapered, and another medication should be tried.

Administration Guidelines

- Dissolve 25 or 40 units of ACTH in 1 or 2 mL of NS injection or sterile water for injection. The solution is stable for 24 hours at room temperature or for 1 week under refrigeration.
- If using the repository suspension, warm to room temperature before administration. Shake thoroughly prior to administration.
- Using a 22-gauge needle, inject deeply into a large muscle mass (IM). Aspirate prior to injection to avoid injection into a blood vessel. Massage area following administration. Rotate sites of injection.

Patient Education

1. Adverse effects that you should report to your physician as soon as possible include:
    bloody or black, tarry stools
    nausea, vomiting
    stomach pain
    rounding out of face
    weight gain, increased thirst
    frequent passing of urine
    fever, sore throat, sneezing, cough, or other signs of infection
    wounds that will not heal
    confusion, excitement, restlessness
    depression, mood swings
    irregular heartbeat
    pain in hips, back, ribs, arms, shoulders, or legs
    pain, redness, swelling, signs of allergy, or scarring at the injection site

skin problems, acne, thin and shiny skin
swelling of feet or lower legs
unusual bruising, pinpoint red spots on the skin
unusual tiredness or weakness.

2. Avoid contact with people who have an infection. You will have an increased risk of infection while receiving corticotropin. Do not receive any vaccinations as you may get a strong reaction. Avoid people who have recently taken the oral polio vaccine. Tell your physician if you are exposed to anyone with measles or chickenpox, or if you develop sores or blisters that do not heal properly.

3. If you are going to have surgery, tell your physician that you have received corticotropin within the last 12 months.

See Box 2.7 and Box 2.8.

Box 2.7 Relative Contraindications to Use of Corticotropin (ACTH)

- Adrenal insufficiency
- Cushing syndrome
- Hypercortisolism
- Heart failure
- Herpes infection
- Ocular infections
- Porcine protein hypersensitivity
- Scleroderma
- Surgery

Box 2.8 Corticotropin (ACTH) Precautions

- Corticosteroid hypersensitivity
- Diabetes mellitus
- Hypothyroidism
- Hepatic diseases
- Hypernatremia
- Hypertension
- Hypokalemia
- Renal diseases
- Infections
- Myasthenia gravis
- Thromboembolic diseases

See Chapters 12–14.

Eslicarbazepine acetate

Brand Name: Aptiom®.

Dosage Forms: Tablets 200, 400, 600, 800 mg.

Dosage

Starting Dose: 400 mg orally once daily for one week.

Maintenance Dose: The usual maintenance dose is 800 mg once daily.

Maximum Dosage Limit: 1200 mg/day.

Discontinuation Schedule: A dosage reduction of 20–25% per 1–2 weeks is a safe discontinuation regimen.

Administration Guidelines

May be taken with or without food. The Aptiom® tablet may be crushed or swallowed whole.

Patient Education

1. If you miss a dose, take it as soon as you can. If it is almost time for your next dose, take only that dose. Do not take double or extra doses.
2. Side effects that you should report to your physician as soon as possible include

    suicidal behavior and ideation

    new or worse depression, anxiety, irritability or changes in behavior or mood

    hives; difficult breathing; swelling of your face, lips, tongue, or throat

    nausea

    lack of energy, feeling tired or irritable, severe weakness

    muscle pain

    confusion, vision changes, thinking problems,

    trouble with walking or coordination

    upper stomach pain, loss of appetite, dark urine, jaundice.
3. Do not stop taking your medicine suddenly. Your physician may want you to reduce your dose gradually.
4. You may get drowsy. Do not drive, use machinery, or do anything that requires mental alertness until you know how this drug affects you.
5. Report to your physician if you notice any changes.
6. If you are female and are taking birth-control pills, you should know that the birth control might not work as well while you are taking eslicarbazepine. Discuss this issue with your physician.

See Box 2.9 and Box 2.10.

Box 2.9 Contraindications to Use of Eslicarbazepine acetate

• Hypersensitivity to eslicarbazepine acetate or oxcarbazepine

---

Box 2.10 Eslicarbazepine acetate Precautions

• Breastfeeding
• Pregnancy
• Elderly
• Kidney diseases
• Severe liver diseases

See Chapters 9–13.

Ethosuximide

Brand Name: Zarontin®.

Dosage Forms: Capsules 250 mg; Syrup 250 mg/5 mL.

Dosage

Starting Dose

Adults and children >6 years: 250 mg PO 1–3 times daily.

Children 3–6 years: 10–15 mg/kg/day (maximum initial dose 250 mg/day), given in 1–3 divided doses.

Titration and Maintenance Dose

Adults and children >6 years: May increase dosage by 250 mg/day at 4- to 7-day intervals, until seizure control is achieved, or to a maximum dose of 1.5 g/day. The usual maintenance dose is 20–40 mg/kg/day (750–1500 mg/day), given in 2–3 divided doses. *Children 3–6 years:* Increase every 4–7 days; usual maintenance dose is 15–40 mg/kg/day, given in 2–3 divided doses.

Maximum Dosage Limit: Dosages exceeding 1.5 g daily should be administered only under strict supervision.

Discontinuation Schedule: A gradual reduction over 4 weeks is recommended (or 50% per week). If necessary, abrupt discontinuation of ethosuximide is probably safe because of its long half-life.

Administration Guidelines

Take with food or after meals to avoid stomach upset

Contraindication

- *Succinimide hypersensitivity*

Patient Education

1. If you miss a dose, take it as soon as possible. However, if it is within 4 hours of your next dose, skip the missed dose and go back to your regular dosing schedule. Do not use double doses.
2. Side effects that you should report to your physician as soon as possible include:
   chest pain or tightness
   shortness of breath, or wheezing
   fever, sore throat
   mouth ulcers
   mood changes, nervousness, or hostility
   muscle aches
   unusual tiredness or weakness
   redness, blistering, peeling or loosening of the skin, including inside the mouth
   skin rash and itching
   unusual bleeding or bruising.
3. You may get drowsy, dizzy, or have blurred vision. Do not drive, use machinery, or do anything that requires mental alertness until

you know how ethosuximide affects you. To reduce dizzy or fainting spells, do not sit or stand up quickly. Alcohol can increase
drowsiness and dizziness. Avoid alcoholic drinks.
4. If you are going to have surgery, tell your physician that you are
taking ethosuximide.

See Box 2.11.

Box 2.11 Ethosuximide Precautions

- Abrupt discontinuation
- Bone marrow suppression
- Breastfeeding
- Pregnancy
- Infants

- Porphyria
- Hematological diseases
- Renal diseases
- Hepatic diseases

See Chapters 9, 10, 12, 13, and 18.

Methsuximide

Brand Name: Celontin®.

Dosage Forms: Capsules 150, 300 mg.

Administration and Dosage

Adults: 300–600 mg/day in 2–3 divided doses for the first week; may
increase by 300 mg/day at weekly intervals up to 1.5 g/day in 3 divided
doses; an initial maintenance dose of 900 mg/day is advised.

Children: 10–15 mg/kg/day in 3 divided doses; increase weekly up to a
maximum of 30 mg/kg/day.

Ezogabine

Brand Name: Potiga™.

Other names: Retigabine (generic); Trobalt® (brand) in Europe.

Dosage Forms: Tablets 50 mg, 100 mg, 200 mg, 300 mg, and 400 mg.

Dosage

Starting Dose
Adults (>18 years): 300 mg/day in 3 divided doses. In elderly (> 65 years),
150 mg/day in 3 divided doses.

Titration and Maintenance Dose
Adults: Titrate by 150 mg increase per week. Usual maintenance dose
is 200 to 300 mg three times a day (600–900 mg/day). May increase
to 1200 mg/day, in 3 divided doses, based on efficacy and tolerability.
At 1200 mg/day, the incidence of dose-related adverse effects may significantly affect patient tolerance. Because ezogabine may cause retinal

abnormalities with long-term use, patients who fail to show substantial clinical benefit after adequate titration should be discontinued from ezogabine.

Maximum Dosage Limits:
Adults: 1200 mg/day. In elderly (> 65 years), 750 mg/day in 3 divided doses.

Children and adolescents <18 years: Safe and effective use has not been established.

Discontinuation Schedule: If ezogabine dose is reduced, discontinued, or substituted with an alternative medication, the dosage should be gradually reduced over a period of at least 3 weeks, unless safety concerns require abrupt withdrawal.

Administration Guidelines
Should be given orally in 3 equally divided doses daily, with or without food. Tablets should be swallowed whole.

Relative Contraindication
• Hypersensitivity to ezogabine.

Patient Education

1. If you miss a dose, take it as soon as you can. If it is almost time for your next dose, take only that dose. Do not take double or extra doses.
2. You should have a complete eye exam if you are currently taking ezogabine or before starting treatment, and then every 6 months while taking ezogabine.
3. Side effects that you should report to your physician as soon as possible include:
   - inability to start urinating
   - trouble emptying your bladder
   - pain with urination
   - suicidal thinking and behavior
   - hallucinations
   - new or worse depression, anxiety, irritability or changes in behavior or mood
   - loss of coordination
   - vision changes
   - fast, slow, or pounding heartbeat
   - any changes in color to your body
   - rash, itching, swelling, severe dizziness, or trouble breathing.
4. You may get drowsy or dizzy while using ezogabine. Do not drive, use machinery, or do anything that requires mental alertness until you know how ezogabine affects you. Alcohol can increase drowsiness and dizziness. Avoid alcoholic drinks.
5. Do not stop taking ezogabine suddenly.

See Box 2.12.

Box 2.12 Ezogabine Precautions

- Breastfeeding
- Pregnancy
- Elderly
- Hepatic impairment

- Renal impairment
- Heart diseases
- Ocular diseases (eg, retinal abnormalities)

See Chapters 9–12, 16, 17, and 27.

Felbamate

Brand Names: Felbatol®, Taloxa®.

Dosage Forms: Tablets 400 mg, 600 mg; Suspension 600 mg/5 mL.

Dosage

Starting Dose:
Adults and adolescents >14 years: 1200 mg/day in 3 divided doses for monotherapy or adjunctive therapy for the first 2 weeks.

Adolescents and children 2–14 years of age: 15 mg/kg/day in 3 divided doses only as adjunctive therapy for the first 2 weeks.

Titration and Maintenance Dose

Adults and adolescents >14 years: For monotherapy increase 600 mg every 2 weeks under close clinical supervision to 2400 mg/day. Thereafter, increase up to 3600 mg/day based on clinical response. For adjunctive therapy, follow these two steps:

- While starting felbamate, reduce the dosage of present AEDs (phenytoin, phenobarbital, valproic acid, and carbamazepine) by 20%.
- Increase the dosage of felbamate by 1200 mg/day every week up to 3600 mg/day. Further reduction of concomitant AEDs dosage may be necessary.

Adolescents and children 2–14 years of age: For adjunctive therapy, follow these two steps:

- While starting felbamate, reduce the dosage of present AEDs (phenytoin, phenobarbital, valproic acid, and carbamazepine) by 20%.
- Increase the dosage of felbamate by 15 mg/kg/day every week up to 45 mg/ kg/day. Further reduction of concomitant AED dosage may be necessary.

Note: For conversion to monotherapy in adults and adolescents above 14 years of age, follow these four steps:

1. Initiate felbamate at 1200 mg/day in 3–4 divided doses.
2. Reduce the dosage of concomitant AEDs by one third.
3. At week 2, increase felbamate dosage to 2400 mg/day and reduce the dosage of concomitant AEDs by an additional one third of the original doses.

4. At week 3, increase felbamate dosage to 3600 mg/day and reduce the dosage or discontinue other AEDs as clinically indicated.

Note: Loading dose is not recommended.

Note: The elderly may require lower initial doses of felbamate and slower dose titration.

Maximum Dosage Limits

Adults and adolescents >14 years: 5400 mg/day (doses >3600 mg/day may be associated with greater risk of aplastic anemia and liver failure).

Adolescents and children 2–14 years of age: 45 mg/kg/day.

Discontinuation Schedule: A dosage reduction of 20%–25% per 2 weeks is safe at the time of discontinuation.

Administration Guidelines

Administer with meals to minimize gastrointestinal side effects.

Patient Education

1. If you miss a dose, take it as soon as you can. If it is almost time for your next dose, take only that dose. Do not take double or extra doses.
2. Side effects that you should report to your physician immediately include
   fainting
   fast or irregular heartbeat
   wheezing or trouble breathing
   skin rash, hives, or itching
   swelling in face, throat, or lips
   unusual bleeding or bruising
   yellow eyes or skin
   loss of seizure control
   unusual tiredness or weakness.
3. Side effects that you should report to your physician as soon as possible include:
   constipation
   loss of appetite, nausea, or vomiting
   fever
   drowsiness or dizziness
   headache
   trouble sleeping, nervousness.
4. Taking felbamate has led to a few cases of a serious blood disorder called aplastic anemia and a few cases of liver failure. Talk to your physician about these risks.
5. Make sure your doctor knows if you have liver or kidney disease or a history of blood problems.
6. You may get drowsy, dizzy, or have blurred vision. Do not drive, use machinery, or do anything that requires mental alertness until you know how felbamate affects you. To reduce dizzy or fainting

spells, do not sit or stand up quickly. Alcohol can increase drowsiness and dizziness. Avoid alcoholic drinks.
7. Felbamate may make your skin more sensitive to the sun or ultra-violet light. Keep out of the sun, or wear protective clothing outdoors and use a sunscreen (at least SPF 15). Do not use sun lamps or sun tanning beds or booths.

See Box 2.13 and Box 2.14.

Box 2.13 Relative Contraindications to Use of Felbamate

- Blood disorders
- Hepatic impairment
- Hypersensitivity to felbamate
- Hypersensitivity to methocarbamol or meprobamate

See Chapters 13 and 18.

Box 2.14 Felbamate Precautions

- Renal impairment
- Breastfeeding
- Pregnancy
- Elderly
- Abrupt discontinuation
- Sunlight or ultraviolet exposure

See Chapters 9–12 and 26.

Gabapentin
Brand Names: Gabarone®, Neurontin®.

Dosage Forms
Gabarone®: Tablets 100 mg, 300 mg, 400 mg.

Gabapentin (Neurontin®): Tablets 600 mg, 800 mg; capsule 100 mg, 300 mg, 400 mg; oral solution 250 mg/5 mL.

Dosage

Starting Dose
Adolescents, adults, and elderly: 300 mg one or two times per day. *Children 3–12 years:* 10–15 mg/kg/day PO in 3 divided doses.

Titration and Maintenance Dose
Adolescents, adults, and elderly: May increase rapidly using 300 mg at bed time on day 1, 300 mg twice daily on day 2, and then 300 mg three times daily starting on day 3. Usual maintenance dose is 900–1800 mg/ day, however doses up to 3600 mg/day have been used. Do not give doses less frequently than every 12 hours. Dosage adjustments of other anticonvulsants are not necessary. Doses for the elderly are often lower and can be based on CrCl.

Children 3–12 years: Titrate upward to effective dose over a period of 3 days. If >5 years, the effective dose is 25–35 mg/kg/day PO, given in 3 divided doses. If 3–4 years of age, the effective dose is 40 mg/kg/day PO, given in 3 divided doses. Do not give doses less frequently than every 12 hours. Depending on the clinical response, titration may continue as needed up to 50 mg/kg/day. Doses higher than 50 mg/kg/day have occasionally been used.

Children <3 years: Safety is not established. However, experts administer it to their patients, whenever benefits outweigh the risks.

Note: Loading dose is not suggested.

Maximum Dosage Limits
Adults, elderly, and adolescents: 3600 mg/day PO (higher doses have been used but are probably not more effective).

Children 3–12 years: 50 mg/kg/day PO suggested; higher dosages occasionally have been used in refractory patients.

Discontinuation Schedule: If gabapentin dose is reduced or discontinued, this should be done gradually over a minimum of 1 week. A dosage reduction of 20%–25% per 2 weeks is safe at the time of discontinuation.

Administration Guidelines
May be administered without regard to meals; however, administration with meals may minimize adverse gastrointestinal effects.

In patients with difficulty in swallowing, gabapentin capsules may be opened and the contents mixed with drinks (eg, orange juice) or foods (eg, applesauce). Scored tablets may be cut in half for dosage titration or ease of swallowing. If the scored 600- or 800-mg tablets are split, the extra half-tablet should be used for the next dose. If the extra half-tablet is not used within 3 days, it should be thrown away.

Contraindication

- *Gabapentin hypersensitivity*

Patient Education

1. If you miss a dose, take it as soon as you can. However, if it is less than 4 hours until your next dose, do not take the missed dose and return to your regular dosing schedule. Do not take double or extra doses.
2. Side effects that you should report to your physician as soon as possible include:
   difficulty breathing or tightening of the throat
   swelling of lips or tongue
   rash
   fever
   hyperactivity
   hostile or aggressive behavior
   mood changes or changes in behavior
   difficulty concentrating

3. You may get drowsy, dizzy, or have blurred vision. Do not drive, use machinery, or do anything that requires mental alertness until you know how gabapentin affects you. To reduce dizzy or fainting spells, do not sit or stand up quickly. Alcohol can increase drowsiness and dizziness. Avoid alcoholic drinks.

4. If you are going to have surgery, tell your physician that you are taking gabapentin.

See Box 2.15.

Box 2.15 Gabapentin Precautions

- Abrupt discontinuation
- Absence seizure
- Breastfeeding
- Pregnancy

- Infants
- Children
- Elderly
- Renal impairment

See Chapters 7 and 9–12.

Lacosamide

Brand Name: Vimpat®.

Dosage Forms: Tablets 50 mg, 100 mg, 150 mg, 200 mg, syrup 10 mg/ml, 200 mg/20 mL injection.

Dosage

Starting Dose
Adolescents >17 years, adults: 100 mg/day in 2 divided doses.

Titration and Maintenance Dose
Adolescents >17 years, adults: Titrate by 100 mg per week. Usual maintenance dose is 200-400 mg per day in 2 divided doses. May increase to 600 mg/day, in 2 divided doses, based on efficacy and tolerability. In clinical trials, the 600 mg daily dose was not more effective than the 400 mg daily dose, and was associated with a substantially higher rate of adverse reactions.

Maximum Dosage Limits: 600 mg/day.

Children <17 years: Safe and effective use has not been established.

Discontinuation Schedule: If lacosamide dose is reduced, discontinued, or substituted with an alternative medication, this should be done gradually over a minimum interval of 1 week.

Administration Guidelines
May be administered without regard to meals.

Note: Lacosamide injection for intravenous use is indicated when oral administration is temporarily not feasible. In this situation, the initial total daily intravenous dosage should be equivalent to the total daily dosage and frequency of oral lacosamide and should be infused intravenously over a period of 30 to 60 minutes. At the end of the intravenous treatment period, the patient may be switched to lacosamide oral administration at the equivalent daily dosage and frequency of the intravenous administration.

Relative Contraindication

- Hypersensitivity to lacosamide

Patient Education

1. If you miss a dose, take it as soon as you can. If it is almost time for your next dose, take only that dose. Do not take double or extra doses.
2. Side effects that you should report to your physician as soon as possible include:
    fast, slow, or pounding heartbeat
    shortness of breath
    feel lightheaded
    fainted
    suicidal behavior and ideation
    new or worse depression, anxiety, irritability or changes in behavior or mood
    rash, itching, swelling, severe dizziness, or trouble breathing.
3. You may get drowsy or dizzy while using lacosamide. Do not drive, use machinery, or do anything that needs mental alertness until you know how lacosamide affects you.
4. Do not stop taking lacosamide suddenly. This medication may cause dependence, especially if it has been used regularly for an extended period of time, or if it has been used in high doses. In such cases, if you suddenly stop this drug, withdrawal reactions may occur.

See Box 2.16.

Box 2.16 Lacosamide Precautions

Suicidal behavior and ideation

Cardiac rhythm and conduction abnormalities

Syncope

Phenylketonuria

Pregnancy

Breastfeeding

Renal impairment

Hepatic impairment

See Chapters 9, 10, 12–14, 17, and 22.

Lamotrigine

Brand Name: Lamictal®.

Dosage Forms

Lamotrigine (Lamictal®): Tablets 25 mg, 100 mg, 150 mg, 200 mg.

Lamotrigine (Lamictal®) chewable dispersible: Chewable tablets 2 mg, 5 mg, 25 mg.

Dosage

In patients not receiving valproic acid or enzyme-inducing AEDs (e.g., carbamazepine, phenobarbital, primidone, phenytoin):

Starting Dose

Adults and adolescents >12 years of age: 25 mg daily for the first 2 weeks.

Children and adolescents 2–12 years of age: 0.3 mg/kg/day in 1 or 2 divided doses given for the first 2 weeks (rounded down to the nearest whole tablet).

Titration and Maintenance Dose

Adults and adolescents >12 years of age: 25 mg twice daily (50 mg/day) for weeks 3–4; then the dose may be increased by up to 50 mg daily every 1–2 weeks until the maintenance dosage is achieved. The usual maintenance dose is 200–400 mg/day, given in 1–2 divided doses.

Children and adolescents 2–12 years of age: 0.6 mg/kg/day given in 2 divided doses for weeks 3–4. Round the dose down to the nearest whole tablet. Thereafter, the dose should be increased every 1–2 weeks as follows: calculate 0.6 mg/kg/day, round this amount down to the nearest whole tablet, and add this amount to the previously administered daily dose. The usual maintenance dose is 4.5–7.5 mg/kg/day (maximum 300 mg/day in 2 divided doses). Maintenance dose in patients less than 30 kg may need to be increased by as much as 50%, based on clinical response.

In patients currently receiving treatment with an enzyme-inducing AED (eg, carbamazepine, phenobarbital, primidone, phenytoin)
Starting Dose

Adults and adolescents >12 years: 50 mg daily for the first 2 weeks.

Children 2–12 years of age: 0.6 mg/kg/day in 2 divided doses given for the first 2 weeks.

Titration and Maintenance Dose

Adults and adolescents >12 years: 100 mg daily is given in two divided doses for weeks 3–4. Thereafter, doses may be increased by 100 mg/day every 1–2 weeks until the maintenance dosage is achieved. The usual maintenance dose is 300–500 mg/day given in 2 divided doses (maximum 700 mg/day in these patients). Conversion to monotherapy, if desired, requires two transitional steps. First, the patient is titrated to the targeted dose of lamotrigine while maintaining the dose of the enzyme-inducing AED at a fixed level. The recommended target maintenance dose for monotherapy conversion is 150–200 mg twice daily (total 300–400 mg daily, although lower doses may be effective). Second, after achieving the targeted lamotrigine dose, the enzyme-inducing AED is gradually withdrawn over a period of 6–12 weeks. If side effects appear after stopping the enzyme-inducing AED, the lamotrigine dose may need to be lowered, because its level will rise as hepatic enzyme activity returns to normal.

Children and adolescents 2–12 years of age: 1.2 mg/kg/day given in 2 divided doses for weeks 3–4. Round the dose down to the nearest whole tablet. After week 4, the usual maintenance dose range is 5–15 mg/kg/day (maximum 400 mg/day) given in 2 divided doses for adjunctive therapy. To achieve the usual maintenance dose, the dose may be increased every 1–2 weeks by about 1.2 mg/kg/day (round this amount down to the nearest whole tablet, and add this amount to the previously administered daily dose). Maintenance doses in patients weighing <30 kg may need to be increased by as much as 50%, based on clinical response. It may take several weeks to months to achieve an individualized maintenance dose.

In patients currently receiving valproic acid with or without enzyme-inducing AEDs or other AEDs concomitantly:
Starting Dose
Adults and adolescents >12 years of age: 25 mg every other day for the first 2 weeks.

Children and adolescents 2–12 years of age: 0.15 mg/kg/day in 1 or 2 divided doses given for the first 2 weeks (rounded down to the nearest whole tablet).

Titration and Maintenance Dose
Adults and adolescents >12 years of age: 25 mg daily for weeks 3–4; then, the dose may be increased by 25–50 mg daily every 2 weeks until the maintenance dosage is achieved. The usual maintenance dose is 100–400 mg/day, given in 1–2 divided doses. The usual maintenance dose range for patients who add lamotrigine to valproic acid alone is 100–200 mg/day.

Children and adolescents 2–12 years of age: 0.3 mg/kg/day given in 1 or 2 divided doses for weeks 3–4. Round the dose down to the nearest whole tablet. After week 4, the usual maintenance dose range is from 1–5 mg/kg/day (maximum 200 mg/day) given in 1 or 2 divided doses. To achieve the usual maintenance dose, doses may be increased every 1–2 weeks by 0.3 mg/kg/day (round this amount down to the nearest whole tablet, and add this amount to the previously administered daily dose). Maintenance doses in patients weighing less than 30 kg may need to be increased by as much as 50%, based on clinical response. The usual maintenance dose range in patients adding lamotrigine to valproic acid alone is 1–3 mg/kg/day.

Note: Conversion to lamotrigine monotherapy from combined lamotrigine and valproate therapy in adults requires 4 steps:

1. The patient should be stabilized on a current maintenance dose of valproate and a target dose of lamotrigine 150–200 mg/day

while taking valproate. If the patient is not currently at lamotrigine 150–200 mg/day, the dose may be increased by 25–50 mg/day every 1–2 weeks to reach that dose.

2. While maintaining lamotrigine dose at 150–200 mg/day, decrease valproate dose to 500 mg/day by decrements of 250–500 mg/day per week and maintain valproate dose of 500 mg/day for 1 week.
3. Increase lamotrigine dose to 300 mg/day while simultaneously decreasing valproate dose to 250 mg/day and maintain for 1 week.
4. Finally, discontinue valproate completely and increase lamotrigine dose as needed for seizure control.

Note: Lamotrigine should be initiated at a low-dose, with gradual increase. This may minimize the occurrence of skin rash.

Note: Avoid use in children weighing <6.7 kg because therapy cannot be initiated using the dosing guidelines and currently available chewable tablet strengths.

Note: If the decision is made to restart a patient who has discontinued lamotrigine for a period of more than 5 half-lives, it is recommended that initial dosing recommendations and guidelines be followed.

Maximum Dosage Limits: Individualize the maximum dosage limits to the patient's age, weight, indication, concurrent medication, and clinical response.

Discontinuation Schedule: Discontinuation of lamotrigine should be done in a stepwise fashion over 2–6 weeks (approximately 50% dosage reduction per week), unless safety concerns warrant a more rapid withdrawal.

Administration Guidelines

May be administered without regard to meals.

Note: The lowest available tablet strength is a 2-mg chewable dispersible tablet, and all doses should be rounded down to the nearest 2-mg dose. Only whole dispersible tablets should be administered; do not cut in half.

Contraindication

- *Hypersensitivity to lamotrigine*

Patient Education

1. If you take regular Lamictal® tablets, swallow the tablets with a drink of water. Do not chew these tablets, as they have a bitter taste. If lamotrigine upsets your stomach, take it with food or milk.
2. Lamictal® chewable dispersible tablets may be swallowed whole, chewed, mixed in water, or mixed in diluted fruit juice to aid swallowing. To mix the tablets in water or juice, add the tablets to a small amount of liquid in a glass or spoon. The tablets will dissolve in about 1 minute. Once dissolved, mix or swirl the liquid, and take

the entire solution immediately. It is important that you swallow all of the liquid used to prepare the dose, so that the full prescribed dose is given.

3. If you miss a dose, take it as soon as you can. If it is almost time for your next dose, take only that dose. Do not take double or extra doses.

4. Side effects that you should report to your physician immediately include:
   fever
   painful sores in the mouth, eyes, or nose
   redness, blistering, peeling or loosening of the skin, including
       inside the mouth
   skin rash of any type, itching
   swelling of the face, lips or tongue
   swollen lymph glands.

5. Side effects you should report to your physician as soon as possible include:
   blurred or double vision
   hand tremor
   somnolence, cognitive difficulties
   uncontrollable eye movements
   changes in seizure type or frequency
   depression or mood changes
   difficulty walking or controlling muscle movements
   unusual weakness or tiredness.

6. You may get drowsy or dizzy or have blurred vision. Do not drive, use machinery, or do anything that requires mental alertness until you know how lamotrigine affects you. To reduce dizzy or fainting spells, do not sit or stand up quickly. Alcohol can increase drowsiness and dizziness. Avoid alcoholic drinks or medicines containing alcohol.

7. If you are female and are taking hormonal birth control methods (eg, birth control pills), you should know that the birth control might not work as well while you are taking lamotrigine. Discuss this issue with your physician.

8. If you are going to have surgery, tell your physician that you are taking lamotrigine.

See Box 2.17.

Box 2.17 Lamotrigine Precautions

- Hypersensitivity to other antiepileptic drugs
- Abrupt discontinuation
- Suicidal ideation
- Pregnancy
- Labor and delivery

- Breastfeeding
- Children
- Elderly
- Hepatic diseases
- Renal impairment

See Chapters 9–13, 22, and 26.

Levetiracetam

Brand Names: Keppra®.

Dosage Forms: Tablets 250 mg, 500 mg, 750 mg, 1000 mg; oral solution 100 mg/mL; injection 500 mg/5 mL.

Dosage

Starting Dose

Adults and adolescents >16 years: 250–500 mg twice daily.

Adolescents and children 4–15 years: 10 mg/kg twice daily (20 mg/kg/day).

Children <4 years: Safe and effective use has not been established. However, experts administer it to their patients whenever benefits outweigh the risks.

Titration and Maintenance Dose

Adults and adolescents >16 years: Usual maintenance dose is 500–750 mg twice daily. May be titrated as needed by 1000 mg/day every 2 weeks until achievement of good clinical response (not to exceed 3000 mg/day), in two divided doses. For conversions between PO and IV administration, use equivalent total daily dosages and frequencies. Doses >3000 mg/day may not provide additional benefit.

Adolescents and children 4–15 years: Increase the daily dose every 2 weeks by increments of 20 mg/kg/day to the recommended dose of 60 mg/kg/day PO twice daily. If a patient cannot tolerate a total daily dose of 60 mg/kg, the daily dose may be reduced. If body weight <20 kg, administer oral solution; if body weight >20 kg, administer either solution or tablets.

Note: Treatment may be initiated with either IV or PO therapy.

Note: Loading dose is not necessary.

Note: Minimum known effective dosage is 1000 mg/day in adults. Lower doses have not been fully tested.

Note: The total daily dose should be the same when switching from oral to IV formulations.

Maximum Dosage Limits *Adolescents >16 years, adults and elderly:* 3000 mg/day PO or IV. *Adolescents <16 years and children:* 60 mg/kg/day PO for the treatment of partial seizures (maximum 3000 mg/day); 3000 mg/day PO for the treatment of myoclonic seizures; IV administration not recommended. *Children 4–11 years:* 60 mg/kg/day PO.

Discontinuation Schedule: A dosage reduction of 20%–25% per 2 weeks is safe at the time of discontinuation.

Administration Guidelines

Oral Administration

- May be administered without regard to meals.
- Tablets are crushable but have a bitter taste.

Intravenous Administration

- Dilute the total dose in 100 mL of compatible diluent (0.9% sodium chloride injection, lactated Ringer's injection, or dextrose 5% injection) and infuse over 15 minutes.
- Diluted preparation is stable for at least 24 hours when stored in polyvinyl chloride bags at controlled room temperature of 15–30°C (59–86°F).
- Diluted preparation is physically compatible with lorazepam, diazepam, and valproate sodium.

Contraindication

- Hypersensitivity to levetiracetam

Patient Education

1. If you miss a dose, take it as soon as you can. If it is almost time for your next dose, take only that dose. Do not take double or extra doses.
2. Side effects that you should report to your physician immediately include
   > difficulty breathing or tightening of the throat
   > rash
   > swelling of lips or tongue.
3. Side effects you should report to your physician as soon as possible include
   > agitation, restlessness, irritability, or other changes in mood
   > changes in seizure type or frequency
   > difficulty walking or controlling muscle movements
   > unusual weakness or tiredness.
4. You may get drowsy or dizzy. Do not drive, use machinery, or do anything that requires mental alertness until you know how levetiracetam affects you. To reduce dizzy spells, do not sit or stand up quickly. Alcohol can increase drowsiness and dizziness. Avoid alcoholic drinks or medicines containing alcohol.
5. If you are going to have surgery, tell your physician that you are taking levetiracetam.

See Box 2.18.

Box 2.18 Levetiracetam Precautions

- Abrupt discontinuation
- Breastfeeding
- Pregnancy
- Children
- Elderly

- Depression
- Psychosis
- Renal diseases
- Renal failure

See Chapters 9–12 and 22.

Oxcarbazepine

Brand Name: Trileptal®.

Dosage Forms: Tablets 150 mg, 300 mg, 600 mg; oral suspension 300 mg/5 mL.

Dosage

Starting Dose:
Adults and adolescents > 16 years: 150–300 mg twice daily.

Adolescents and children 2–16 years: 8–10 mg/kg/day in two divided doses. For patients < 20 kg, a starting dose of 16–20 mg/kg may be considered.

Titration and Maintenance Dose:
Adults and adolescents > 16 years: Oxcarbazepine should be titrated upward by 300–600 mg/day every week over 2 to 4 weeks to achieve the recommended dose of 900–2400 mg/day.

Adolescents and children 2–16 years: Increase the dose by 5 mg/kg/day every three days to the recommended daily maintenance dosage as follows:

- 30–50 mg/kg/day in children 2–4 years of age
- 600–900 mg/day for those 20–24.9 kg
- 900–1200 mg/day for those 25–34.9 kg
- 900–1500 mg/day for those 35–44.9 kg
- 1200–1500 mg/day for those 45–49.9 kg
- 1200–1800 mg/day for those 50–59.9 kg
- 1200–2100 mg/day for those 60–69.9 kg
- 1500–2100 mg/day for those >= 70 kg.

Children and infants < 2 years: Safe and effective use has not been established. However, experts administer it to their patients whenever benefits outweigh the risks.

Note: Loading dose is not studied.

Note: When converting to oxcarbazepine from other AEDs, initiate at 300 mg twice daily while beginning to reduce the dose of other AEDs. The dosage of concurrent AEDs should be completely withdrawn over 3 to 6 weeks as tolerated.

Note: For adjunct treatment of partial seizures with or without secondary generalization, maintenance dose is usually up to 1200 mg/day. Dosages above 1200 mg/day are considered more effective; however, many patients withdraw due to intolerable CNS adverse-effects from combined AED therapy.

For conversion of patients from carbamazepine to oxcarbazepine
Individualize the dosage. The usual daily maintenance dose of oxcarbazepine is approximately 1.5 times that of carbamazepine in adults and 1.2 times that of carbamazepine in the elderly.

Maximum Dosage Limits:

- *Adolescents > 16 years, adults and elderly:* 2400 mg/day.

- *Adolescents and children 4–16 years:* age and weight dependent.
- *Children 2 to < 4 years:* 60 mg/kg/day (in 2 divided doses).

Discontinuation Schedule: A dosage reduction of 20%–25% per two weeks is safe at the time of discontinuation.

Administration Guidelines

May be taken without regard to meals.

Oral suspension: Shake well before each use. To ensure accurate dosage, use calibrated oral syringe provided. Dosage may be mixed in a small glass of water prior to administration if desired. Use within 7 weeks of first opening the bottle.

Contraindication

- *Known hypersensitivity to oxcarbazepine*

Patient Education

1. If you miss a dose, take it as soon as you can. If it is almost time for your next dose, take only that dose. Do not take double or extra doses.
2. Side effects that you should report to your physician as soon as possible include
    fever, rash, muscle aches or pain, hives, or difficulty breathing
    redness, blistering, peeling or loosening of the skin, including inside the mouth
    swelling of the legs and ankles
    vision changes
    infection
    unusual bruising or bleeding
    nausea or vomiting
    confusion
    difficulty speaking or walking
    dizziness
    muscle incoordination
    unexplained tiredness or weakness.
3. You may get drowsy or dizzy when you first start taking this medicine. Do not drive, use machinery, or do anything that requires mental alertness until you know how oxcarbazepine affects you. Alcohol can increase drowsiness and dizziness. Avoid alcoholic drinks.
4. If you are female and are taking birth control pills or using other hormonal birth control methods (like injections), you should know that the birth control might not work as well while you are taking this drug. Talk to your physician about alternatives or use of additional birth control methods while taking this drug.
5. If you are going to have surgery, tell your physician that you are taking oxcarbazepine.

See Box 2.19.

Box 2.19 Oxcarbazepine Precautions

- Carbamazepine hypersensitivity
- Breastfeeding
- Pregnancy
- Infants
- Elderly
- Abrupt discontinuation

See Chapters 9–12, 14, and 26.

- Ethanol intoxication
- Hyponatremia
- Heart failure
- Cardiac conduction disturbances
- Renal impairment

Perampanel

Brand Name: Fycompa™.

Dosage Forms: Tablets 2 mg, 4 mg, 6 mg, 8 mg, 10 mg, 12 mg.

Dosage

Starting Dose

Children >12 years and adults: 2 mg once daily at bedtime in patients not on enzyme-inducing antiepileptic drugs (AEDs) and 4 mg in patients on enzyme-inducing AEDs.

Titration and Maintenance Dose

Children >12 years and adults: May increase based on clinical response and tolerability by a maximum of 2 mg once daily at bedtime in weekly increments to a dose of 4 mg to 12 mg once daily at bedtime. A dose of 12 mg once daily resulted in somewhat greater reductions in seizure rates than the dose of 8 mg once daily but with a substantial increase in adverse reactions. For elderly, maximum frequency for dosage increases is every two weeks. In patients with mild and moderate hepatic impairment, maximum recommended daily dose is 6 mg and 4 mg once daily at bedtime, respectively; maximum frequency for dosage increases is every two weeks.

Maximum Dosage Limits:
Children >12 years and adults: 12 mg/day.

Children <12 years: Safe and effective use has not been established.

Discontinuation Schedule: If perampanel dose is reduced, discontinued, or substituted with an alternative medication, this should be done gradually, but if withdrawal is a response to adverse events, prompt withdrawal can be considered.

Administration Guidelines
May be administered without regard to meals.

Relative Contraindication

- Hypersensitivity to perampanel

Patient Education

1. Perampanel is usually taken 1 time a day at bedtime.
2. If you miss a dose resume dosing the following day at your pre-scribed daily dose. Do not take double or extra doses.
3. Side effects that you should report to your physician as soon as possible include:
   suicidal thinking and behavior
   new or worse depression, anxiety, irritability or changes in behavior or mood
   dizziness
   gait disturbance
   loss of coordination
   falls
   somnolence and fatigue
   rash, itching, swelling, severe dizziness, or trouble breathing.
4. You may get drowsy or dizzy while using perampanel. Do not drive, use machinery, or do anything that requires mental alertness until you know how perampanel affects you. Alcohol can increase drowsiness and dizziness. Avoid alcoholic drinks.
5. Do not stop taking perampanel suddenly.
6. If you are female and are taking birth control pills, you should know that the birth control might not work as well while you are taking perampanel. Discuss this issue with your physician.

See Box 2.20.

Box 2.20 Perampanel Precautions

- Breastfeeding
- Pregnancy
- Suicidal behavior and ideation
- Elderly
- Central nervous system depression
- Ethanol intoxication

- Hepatic impairment
- Renal impairment

See Chapters 9–13 and 22.

Phenobarbital

Brand Name: Luminal®.

Dosage Forms: Tablets 15 mg, 30 mg, 32 mg, 60 mg, 90 mg, 100 mg; capsules 16 mg (Solfoton®); elixir 15 mg/5 mL, 20 mg/5 mL; injection 30 mg/mL, 60 mg/mL, 65 mg/mL, 130 mg/mL.

Dosage

For the treatment of status epilepticus

Loading Dose (adults, children, and infants): 10–20 mg/kg IV (not to exceed 100 mg/min or 2 mg/kg/min in children). In the absence of mechanical ventilation, a dose of 10 mg/kg IV should be administered initially and followed by an additional 5 mg/kg IV approximately 30–60 minutes after the first dose. An additional 5 mg/kg may be given for refractory seizures. The usual maximum total loading dose is 25–30 mg/kg. A post-distribution serum concentration can be obtained 1–2 hours after completion of the loading infusion to assess the adequacy of the dose. In recent years, it has been our practice to load with 10 mg/kg and then use pentobarbital to avoid a more prolonged coma.

Maintenance Dose: Initiate maintenance dose 12–24 hours after the loading dose. Adverse reactions (eg, apnea, hypotension) may complicate acute seizure management when phenobarbital is given after benzodiazepines (eg, lorazepam or diazepam). Phenobarbital is usually only used when benzodiazepines and phenytoin fail to abort status.

Neonates: Initially, a loading dose of 15–20 mg/kg IV in single or divided doses. In the absence of mechanical ventilation, a smaller dose (10 mg/kg) should be administered initially and followed by an additional dose approximately 30–60 minutes after the first dose. Total loading doses up to 40 mg/kg have been used.

Note: IV benzodiazepines, (eg, lorazepam or diazepam) should be given initially before using barbiturates in most cases.

For the treatment of all types of seizure disorders, including partial seizures, clonic seizures, myoclonic seizures, tonic seizures, or tonic-clonic seizures not responding to other anticonvulsants:

Oral maintenance dosage (also may be given IM or IV if needed):

Adults and adolescents: start at 0.5 mg/kg/day (30 mg at bedtime for typical adult) and titrate in 30 mg increments per 1–2 weeks to total of 1.5–4 mg/kg/day in 1–2 divided doses. Because phenobarbital is sedating and has a long half-life, a single daily dose administered at bedtime is recommended. If morning sedation occurs, then twice daily dosing can be used, with the larger dose at bedtime.

Children 5–12 years: start at 1–2 mg/kg/day and titrate to 3–6 mg/kg/day PO in 1–2 divided doses.

Children 1–5 years: start at 1–2 mg/kg/day and titrate to 6–8 mg/kg/day PO in 1–2 divided doses.

Infants: start at 2 mg/kg/day and titrate to 5–6 mg/kg/day PO in 1–2 divided doses.

Neonates: 1–4 mg/kg PO once daily. May increase to 5 mg/kg/day PO if serum concentrations are inadequate.

Note: Phenobarbital should be titrated upward gradually over several weeks or more to allow patients to develop tolerance to sedative effect. The dosage should be adjusted, as necessary, to achieve a therapeutic phenobarbital concentration (usually 15–40 µg/mL). IV administration should be used only in patients unable to take oral medication.

Note: Oral loading dose is possible as 10–20 mg/kg divided into equal doses and given over 24–48 hours.

Maximum Dosage Limits

Adolescents, adults, and elderly: 300 mg/day PO, provided not sedated at lower doses. *Children and infants:* Individualized dosage.

Discontinuation Schedule: A dosage reduction of 20%–25% per month is safe at the time of discontinuation. Slow taper is advised.

Administration Guidelines

Oral Administration

- All dosage forms may be given with food.
- For patients with difficulty swallowing, tablets may be crushed and mixed with food or fluids.
- Administer undiluted or mixed oral solution with water, milk, or fruit juice. Administer using a calibrated measuring device for accurate measurement of the dose.

Parenteral Administration

- Phenobarbital is administered intramuscularly or intravenously. Intravenous administration is for hospitalized patients only.
- Never inject intra-arterially.
- Protect injection from light.
- Phenobarbital sodium injection is incompatible with many other injectable medications.

Intramuscular (IM) Injection

- Inject deeply into the gluteal muscle to minimize tissue irritation. Do not inject >5 mL into any one site. Aspirate prior to injection to avoid injection into a blood vessel.

Slow Intravenous (IV) Injection

- IV injection should only be used in emergency situations or when other routes are not feasible.
- Avoid extravasation.
- In adult patients, the maximum rate of slow IV injection is 60 mg/min in less-acute situations and a maximum of 100 mg/min for status epilepticus, but hypotension or the need for assisted ventilation

may occur when the drug is administered at these rates. If hypotension occurs, the administration rate should be reduced by 50%. During injection, blood pressure, respiration, and cardiac function should be maintained, vital signs monitored, and equipment for resuscitation and artificial ventilation should be readily available.

- In pediatric patients, phenobarbital should be diluted with at least an equal volume of a compatible fluid and slowly injected at a rate no greater than 2 mg/kg/min in infants and usually no more than 30 mg/min in older children. If hypotension occurs, the administration rate should be reduced by 50%.

Patient Education

1. Try not to miss doses. If you are on a regular schedule and miss a dose, take it as soon as you can. If it is almost time for your next dose, take only that dose. Do not take double or extra doses.
2. Side effects that you should report to your physician as soon as possible include:
   bone tenderness
   changes in the frequency or severity of seizures
   confusion, agitation
   changes in behavior, mood, or mental ability
   hallucinations (seeing and hearing things that are not really there)
   difficulty breathing or shortness of breath
   eye problems
   fever, sore throat
   lightheadedness or fainting spells
   redness, blistering, peeling or loosening of the skin, including inside the mouth
   skin rash, itching, hives
   slow heartbeat
   swelling of the face or lips
   unusual bleeding or bruising, pinpoint red spots on the skin
   weight loss
   yellowing of skin or eyes
   unusual tiredness or weakness.
3. After receiving phenobarbital, you may get drowsy or dizzy. Do not drive, use machinery, or do anything that requires mental alertness until you know how phenobarbital affects you. To reduce dizzy or fainting spells, do not sit or stand up quickly. Alcohol can increase possible unpleasant effects. Avoid alcoholic drinks.
4. Phenobarbital can reduce the effectiveness of birth control pills or other hormonal birth control drugs. Talk to your physician about alternatives or use of additional birth control methods while taking this drug.
5. If you are going to have surgery, tell your physician that you are taking phenobarbital.

See Box 2.21 and Box 2.22.

Box 2.21 Relative Contraindications to Use of Phenobarbital

- Agranulocytosis
- Barbiturate hypersensitivity
- Ethanol intoxication
- Hepatic encephalopathy
- Intra-arterial administration
- Porphyria
- Subcutaneous administration

See Chapters 13, 14, and 18.

Box 2.22 Phenobarbital Precautions

- Intravenous administration
- Carbamazepine hypersensitivity
- Hydantoin hypersensitivity
- Breastfeeding
- Pregnancy
- Labor
- Neonates
- Elderly
- Central nervous system depression and mental status changes
- Depression
- Suicidal ideation
- Substance abuse
- Alcoholism
- Pain
- Osteomalacia/osteoporosis
- Cardiac diseases
- Hypotension
- Anticoagulant therapy
- Hepatic diseases
- Pulmonary diseases
- Sleep apnea
- Renal impairment
- Anuria
- Shock
- Exfoliative dermatitis
- Abrupt discontinuation

See Chapters 6, 9–13, 14, 17, 22, 26, and 29.

Primidone

Brand Name: Mysoline®.

Dosage Forms: Tablets 50 mg, 250 mg; oral suspension 250 mg/5 mL.

Dosage

Starting Dose

Adults, adolescents, and children >8 years: 62.5–250 mg/day once daily at bedtime or divided in 2 doses.

Children <8 years and infants: 50 mg/day at bedtime or divided in 2 doses.

Titration and Maintenance Dose

Adults, adolescents, and children >8 years: Increase dose by 100–125 mg/day every 3–7 days. The usual dose is 750–1500 mg/day in 3–4 divided doses. *Children <8 years and infants:* Increase dose by 50 mg/day every 3–7 days. Usual doses range from 10–25 mg/kg/day in 3–4 divided doses.

Neonates: 12–25 mg/kg/day in 2–4 divided doses. Start at lower doses and titrate.

Maximum Dosage Limits: *Children >8 years, adolescents, adults and elderly:* 2000 mg/day. *Infants and children <8 years:* 25 mg/kg/day (or up to a maximum dosage 1000 mg/day). *Neonates:* 25 mg/kg/day.

Discontinuation Schedule: A dosage reduction of 20%–25% per month is safe at the time of discontinuation.

Administration Guidelines

Primidone is administered orally with meals to minimize indigestion or gastrointestinal irritation.

Contraindications/Precautions

Because primidone is metabolized to phenobarbital, it shares all the contraindications/precautions of this drug.

Primidone is not commonly used as an anticonvulsant in young children and infants. Due to immature hepatic and renal function (particularly in the first few weeks of life), neonates (especially those with prematurity) must be carefully monitored during primidone use via serum concentrations and clinical status. Children are more likely than adults to react with paradoxical excitement to primidone or to have drug intolerance.

Patient Education

1. If you miss a dose, take it as soon as you can if it is more than an hour until your next dose. If it is almost time for your next dose, take only that dose. Do not take double or extra doses.
2. Side effects that you should report to your physician as soon as possible include
    blurred or double vision, uncontrollable rolling or movements of the eyes
    irritability or mood changes
    unusual excitement or restlessness (more likely in children and the elderly)
    lightheadedness or fainting spells
    shortness of breath or difficulty breathing
    redness, blistering, peeling or loosening of the skin, including inside the mouth
    skin rash, or itching
    unusual weakness or tiredness or sedation.

3. After taking primidone you may get drowsy or dizzy. Do not drive, use machinery, or do anything that requires mental alertness until you know how primidone affects you. To reduce dizzy or fainting spells, do not sit or stand up quickly. Alcohol can increase possible unpleasant effects. Avoid alcoholic drinks.

4. Primidone can reduce the effectiveness of birth control pills or other hormonal birth control drugs. Talk to your physician about alternatives or use of additional birth control methods while taking this drug.

5. If you are going to have surgery, tell your physician that you are taking primidone.

Phenytoin

Brand Names: Dilantin®, Phenytek®.

Dosage Forms: Chewable tablet 50 mg; capsule 100 mg; XR capsule 30 mg, 100 mg, 200 mg, 300 mg; oral suspension 125 mg/5 mL; injection 50 mg/mL.

Note: Intravenous phenytoin solutions contain phenytoin sodium, which is 92% phenytoin. Phenytoin capsules contain phenytoin sodium, which is 92% phenytoin. Chewable tablets and suspensions contain 100% phenytoin. Different phenytoin dosage forms are not directly interchangeable.

Dosage

Intravenous Loading Dosage (in status epilepticus)
Adults, adolescents, children, and infants: Loading dose of 18–20 mg/kg via slow IV push or via IV infusion in NS in patients with unknown or undetectable phenytoin concentrations. In patients with detectable serum phenytoin, reduce loading dose correspondingly. If seizures are not terminated after the initial loading dose, consider additional AEDs. The full antiepileptic effect of phenytoin is not immediate; IV benzodiazepines (eg, lorazepam or diazepam) should be given initially or concurrently. Some experts advocate an additional phenytoin dose of 5–10 mg/kg IV if the initial loading dose fails to terminate seizures (but not in neonates). Total loading dose should not exceed 30 mg/kg. Ideally, begin maintenance dose within 8 hours.

Note: In patients currently receiving phenytoin with suboptimal serum concentrations calculate the required loading dose as follows:

Loading dose = 0.8 × weight × (desired serum level − current serum level)

Loading Dose in Non-Emergent Situations

- Oral non-emergent loading dosage (suspension, chewable tablets, or non-sustained release capsules)

Adults and children: 15–20 mg/kg PO for non-emergent loading doses in a patient not currently on phenytoin. The loading dose can be divided into two doses separated by 2 hours, but it may be given at once in a single dose. Do not use the oral loading dose in emergent situations. Although loading doses of phenytoin have been administered successfully via the oral route, this approach requires several hours to achieve a therapeutic concentration. Sustained-release capsules should not be used for loading doses. In patients with detectable but subtherapeutic serum phenytoin levels, reduce the loading dose correspondingly. Following the completion of oral loading, begin maintenance dose within 12–24 hours.

Note: There is one report of oral phenytoin loading with a single dose of 18 mg/kg capsules or suspension in 44 patients. The drug was well tolerated and mean serum phenytoin level was 15.1 mg/L after 16–24 hours (Osborn et al., 1987).

- Intravenous Non-Emergent Loading Dosage

Adults and children: If the patient cannot take oral doses, IV phenytoin injection could be used following a similar dosing strategy as for oral non-emergent treatment to raise phenytoin serum concentrations. Follow IV administration guidelines.

Titration and Maintenance Dose

Adults: 4.5–7 mg/kg/day PO (may be given IV if needed) is appropriate for most patients. Give phenytoin injection in multiple daily doses, at regular intervals. If sustained-release capsules are used, the dose can be given as a single daily oral dose in many patients once dosage is stabilized. If chewable tablets, oral suspension, or non-sustained-release capsules are used, the daily dosage should be divided into 2–3 divided doses per day. Multiple daily doses should be given at regular intervals. Dosage adjustment for phenytoin is complex due to nonlinear kinetics. If plasma concentration at steady state is <8 µg/mL, the daily dose can be increased by 100 mg/day in adults. If plasma concentration at steady state is >7 and <12 µg/mL, the daily dose can be increased by 50 mg/day, if an increase in level is needed. If plasma concentration at steady state is >11 µg/mL, the daily dose can be increased by 25–30 mg/day in adults if further increase in level is needed. *Adolescents, children, infants, and neonates:* Initially, 5 mg/kg/day PO (IV if needed) in 2 divided doses and adjust to clinical effect and serum drug concentrations. Usual doses range as follows:

- 5–8 mg/kg/day in neonates
- 8–10 mg/kg/day in children 6 months–3 years
- 7.5–9 mg/kg/day in children 4–6 years
- 7–8 mg/kg/day in children 7–9 years
- 6–7 mg/kg/day children 10–16 years

Dosing frequency may be variable in children due to fast drug clearance. Some neonates may require phenytoin every 8 hours.

Note: Monitor phenytoin serum concentrations during chronic therapy.

For seizure prophylaxis due to specific conditions:

1. During neurosurgery
Adults, adolescents, and children: The loading dose is 18–20 mg/kg via IV infusion in NS. Typical initial maintenance dose is 4.5–7 mg/kg/day IV, divided into 2 or more doses as long as needed.

2. In women with pregnancy-induced hypertension
Adult females: 18 mg/kg IV infusion loading dose then daily maintenance as long as needed (delayed-release capsules). Magnesium sulfate is the preferred agent in these patients.

3. For the prophylaxis and treatment of seizures secondary to eclampsia
Adult females: 18 mg/kg IV loading dose followed by daily maintenance as long as needed. Magnesium sulfate is the preferred agent in these patients. In addition, maternal and neonatal morbidity are lower with magnesium.

Maximum Dosage Limits: None. Phenytoin dosage must be individualized.

Discontinuation Schedule: A dosage reduction of 20%–25% per 1–2 weeks is safe at the time of discontinuation.

Administration Guidelines

- Shake oral suspension well prior to each dose. Administer using a calibrated measuring device. If given via an enteral tube, adsorption to the tubing can be minimized by diluting the suspension with a compatible diluent (eg, at least 20 mL of NS or sterile water for administration to adults) before administering. After administration, flush the tube with at least 20 mL of the diluent (in adults). Continuous enteral feedings interfere with phenytoin absorption and lower serum phenytoin concentrations by up to 80% in some patients. Tube feedings should generally be discontinued for 1–2 hours before and after administration of each phenytoin dose.
- For patients with difficulty swallowing, the prompt-release capsules may be opened and the contents mixed with food or fluids. To prevent direct contact with the oral mucosa, the patient should drink a liquid first, followed by the drug mixture and then followed with a full glass of water or milk.
- Administer extended-release capsules intact. Do not crush, cut, or chew. While food does not affect the absorption of Dilantin® Kapseals®, some generic products exhibit reduced absorption in the presence of a high-fat meal. It may be best to administer generic extended-release phenytoin capsules on an empty stomach or in a consistent manner in relation to food to avoid bioavailability problems.
- Do not administer phenytoin by IM injection. IM phenytoin absorption is unreliable and phenytoin may cause tissue injury, necrosis, or aseptic abscess.

- Prior to IV administration, the patient should preferably have good intravenous access. The vein utilized should be free from injury or thrombophlebitis.
- Continuous monitoring of the electrocardiogram, blood pressure, and respiration is essential during loading dose administration and the patient should be observed throughout the period where maximal serum phenytoin concentrations occur, up to 1 hour after the end of a loading dose infusion. In the case of parenteral administration of maintenance doses, continuous clinical cardiac monitoring (rate, rhythm, blood pressure) and close clinical observation are recommended during dose administration.
- Phenytoin IV injections or infusions should be administered through a free-flowing IV of NS or other non-dextrose-containing saline IV solution.
- Avoid extravasation, phenytoin is irritating to tissues and may cause injury.
- The rate of administration of IV phenytoin is critically important. Do not exceed recommended infusion rates:

Adults: Inject IV at a rate not to exceed 50 mg/min. Consider slower infusion rates in those with concurrent cardiac disease.

Elderly or debilitated adults: Inject IV at a rate not to exceed 25–50 mg/ min.

Children: Inject IV at a rate of 0.5–1 mg/kg/min, not to exceed 50 mg/ min. However, the higher infusion rate may be indicated in selected circumstances.

Infants and neonates: Inject IV at a rate not to exceed 0.5–1 mg/kg/min. Due to their small veins, infants may be more at risk of thrombophlebitis or other tissue injury from the use of phenytoin IV. Do not infuse via scalp veins.

- For intermittent IV infusion, dilute phenytoin in NS to a final concentration of ≥6.7 mg/mL. For example: A dosage of 1000 mg would be diluted with NS to a minimum volume of 150 mL.
- Phenytoin injection is poorly soluble; complete infusion administration within 1 hour of infusion preparation.
- Flush the IV line or catheter with NS for injection before and after dose to reduce risk of local vein irritation.

Patient Education

1. Try not to miss a scheduled dosage, especially if you are taking phenytoin extended-release capsules just once per day. If you miss a dose, take it as soon as you can. If it is less than 4 hours to your next dose, take only that dose. If you only take a dose once a day and do not remember until the next day, skip the missed dose and resume your normal schedule. Do not take double or extra doses.

2. Side effects that you should report to your physician as soon as possible include:

> chest pain or tightness
> fast or irregular heartbeat
> fainting spells or lightheadedness
> difficulty breathing, wheezing or shortness of breath
> confusion, nervousness, hostility, or other behavioral changes
> headache
> loss of seizure control
> poor control of body movements or difficulty walking
> dark yellow or brown urine
> vomiting
> yellowing of the eyes or skin
> double vision or uncontrollable and rapid eye movement
> fever, sore throat
> mouth ulcers
> redness, blistering, peeling or loosening of the skin or inside the mouth
> skin rash, itching
> stomach pain
> swollen or painful lymph glands (nodes)
> unusual bleeding or bruising, pinpoint red spots on skin
> sexual problems (painful erections, loss of sexual desire)
> unusual tiredness or weakness.

3. Do not change brands or dosage forms of phenytoin without discussing the change with your physician.

4. You may feel dizzy or drowsy. Do not drive, use machinery, or do anything that requires mental alertness until you know how phenytoin affects you. To reduce the risk of dizzy or fainting spells, do not sit or stand up quickly. Alcohol can make you dizzier. Avoid alcoholic drinks.

5. Birth control pills or other hormonal birth control drugs may not work properly while you are taking phenytoin; talk with your physician about the use of other methods of birth control.

6. Phenytoin can cause unusual growth of gum tissue. Visit your dentist regularly. Problems can arise if you need dental work, and in the daily care of your teeth. Try to avoid damage to your teeth and gums when you brush or floss your teeth.

7. Do not take antacids at the same time as phenytoin. If you get an upset stomach and want to take an antacid or medicine for diarrhea, make sure there is an interval of 2–3 hours before or after you take phenytoin.

8. If you are going to have surgery, tell your physician that you are taking phenytoin.

See Box 2.23 and Box 2.24.

Box 2.23 Relative Contraindications to Use of Phenytoin

- Adams-Stokes syndrome
- Atrioventricular block or bundle-branch block
- Bradycardia
- Bone marrow suppression
- Hydantoin hypersensitivity
- Intramuscular administration
- Jaundice
- Methemoglobinemia

See Chapters 13, 17, and 18.

Box 2.24 Phenytoin Precautions

- Intravenous administration
- Abrupt discontinuation
- Barbiturate hypersensitivity
- Carbamazepine hypersensitivity
- Absence seizures
- Myoclonic seizures
- Breastfeeding
- Pregnancy
- Obstetric delivery
- Neonates
- Elderly
- Psychosis
- Alcoholism
- Dental diseases
- Encephalopathy
- Fever
- Hemolytic anemia
- Lymphoma
- Hodgkin disease
- Cardiac arrhythmias
- Coronary artery disease
- Heart failure
- Hypotension
- Hepatic diseases
- Vitamin K deficiency
- Renal diseases
- Diabetes mellitus
- Thyroid diseases
- Hypoglycemia
- Hyponatremia
- Myasthenia gravis
- Osteomalacia/osteoporosis
- Porphyria
- Radiation therapy
- Systemic lupus erythematosus

See Chapters 7, 9–18, 22, 26, and 29.

Fosphenytoin Sodium

Brand Name: Cerebyx®.

Dosage Forms: 150 mg/2ml (100 mg phenytoin sodium equivalent), 750 mg/10ml (500 mg phenytoin sodium equivalent).

Dosage (PE [Phenytoin Equivalent])

Status Epilepticus: The loading dose of 18–20 mg PE/kg administered at 100–150 mg PE/min.

Non-Emergent and Maintenance Dosing

Loading dose: 15–20 mg PE/kg given IV or IM. Max IV infusion rate is 150 mg PE/minute. In children, rates of infusion should be 1–3 PE/kg/minute.

Maintenance dose: 4–6 mg PE/kg/day.

Administration Guidelines

The dose, concentration, and infusion rate of IV fosphenytoin are expressed as phenytoin sodium equivalent (PE). Dilute fosphenytoin in 5% dextrose or 0.9% saline solution for injection to a concentration range of 1.5–25 mg PE/mL. Intramuscular administration may be given as a single daily dose.

Pregabalin

Brand Name: Lyrica®.

Dosage Forms: Capsules 25 mg, 50 mg, 75 mg, 100 mg, 150 mg, 200 mg, 225 mg, 300 mg.

Dosage

Starting Dose

Children >12 years, adults, and the elderly (CrCl >60 mL/min): 150 mg/day in 2 or 3 divided doses.

Titration and Maintenance Dose

Children >12 years, adults, and the elderly (CrCl >60 mL/min): Titrate by 75 mg to 150 mg per week. Usual maintenance dose is 150 mg twice daily. May increase to 600 mg/day, in 2–3 divided doses, based on efficacy and tolerability. At 600 mg/day, the incidence of dose-related adverse effects (dizziness, drowsiness, and blurred vision) may significantly affect patient tolerance.

Note: Loading dose is not studied.

Maximum Dosage Limits:

Children >12 years, adults, and the elderly: 600 mg/day.

Children <12 years: Safe and effective use has not been established.

Discontinuation Schedule: If pregabalin dose is reduced, discontinued, or substituted with an alternative medication, this should be done gradually over a minimum interval of 1 week.

Administration Guidelines

May be administered without regard to meals.

Relative Contraindication

- Abrupt discontinuation

Patient Education

1. Swallow the capsules with a drink of water. If pregabalin upsets your stomach, take it with food or milk.

2. If you miss a dose, take it as soon as you can. If it is almost time for your next dose, take only that dose. Do not take double or extra doses.
3. Side effects that you should report to your physician as soon as possible include

   change in amount of urine
   slow or irregular heartbeat
   difficulty speaking
   loss of coordination
   mental or mood changes
   uncontrolled movements (eg, tremor, twitching)
   vision changes
   muscle pain/tenderness/weakness (especially if your are tired
       or have a fever)
   stomach/abdominal pain
   unusual bleeding or bruising
   rash, itching, swelling, severe dizziness, or trouble breathing.
4. You may get drowsy or dizzy while using pregabalin. Do not drive, use machinery, or do anything that requires mental alertness until you know how pregabalin affects you. To reduce dizzy or fainting spells, do not sit or stand up quickly. Alcohol can increase drowsiness and dizziness. Avoid alcoholic drinks.
5. If you have a heart condition, such as congestive heart failure, and notice that you are retaining water (edema) and have swelling in your hands or feet, contact your physician immediately.
6. Do not stop taking pregabalin suddenly. This medication may cause dependence, especially if it has been used regularly for an extended period of time, or if it has been used in high doses. In such cases, if you suddenly stop this drug, withdrawal reactions may occur.
7. If you are going to have surgery, tell your physician that you are taking pregabalin.

See Box 2.25.

Box 2.25 Pregabalin Precautions

- Breastfeeding
- Pregnancy
- Infants and children
- Elderly
- Central nervous system depression
- Ethanol intoxication

- Substance abuse
- Heart failure
- Myopathy
- Ocular diseases (e.g., glaucoma)
- Diabetes mellitus
- Renal impairment

See Chapters 9–12, 16, 17, and 27.

Rufinamide

Brand Name: Banzel®.

Dosage Forms: Tablets 100 mg, 200 mg, 400 mg, oral suspension 40 mg/ml.

Dosage

Starting Dose

Children >4 years: 10 mg/kg/day administered in two equally divided doses.

Adults: 400-800 mg/day administered in two equally divided doses.

Note: The safety and effectiveness in patients with Lennox-Gastaut syndrome have not been established in children less than 4 years.

Note: Patients on valproate should begin rufinamide at a dose lower than 10 mg/kg/day (children) or 400 mg/day (adults).

Titration and Maintenance Dose

Children >4 years: Titrate by 10 mg/kg increments every other day to a target dose of 45 mg/kg/day or 3200 mg/day, whichever is less.

Adults: The dose should be increased by 400-800 mg every other day until a maximum dose of 3200 mg/day.

Maximum Dosage Limits:

Children >4 years: 45 mg/kg/day or 3200 mg/day, whichever is less.

Adults: 3200 mg/day.

Discontinuation Schedule: If rufinamide dose is reduced, discontinued, or substituted with an alternative medication, this should be done gradually (25% every 2 days).

Administration Guidelines

Should be given with food. Tablets can be administered whole, as half tablets, or crushed.

Contraindication

- Patients with Familial Short QT syndrome.

Patient Education

1. If you miss a dose, take it as soon as you can. If it is almost time for your next dose, take only that dose. Do not take double or extra doses.
2. Side effects that you should report to your physician as soon as possible include
   loss of coordination
   suicidal thinking and behavior
   severe muscle pain
   unusual bleeding or bruising
   rash, itching, swelling, fever, severe dizziness, or trouble breathing.

3. You may get drowsy or dizzy while using rufinamide. Do not drive, use machinery, or do anything that needs mental alertness until you know how rufinamide affects you. Alcohol can increase drowsiness and dizziness. Avoid alcoholic drinks.
4. Do not stop taking rufinamide suddenly.
5. If you are female and are taking birth control pills, you should know that the birth control might not work as well while you are taking rufinamide. Discuss this issue with your physician.

See Box 2.26.

Box 2.26 Rufinamide Precautions

- Breastfeeding
- Pregnancy
- Hepatic impairment
- Elderly
- Heart diseases

See Chapters 9-11, 13, and 17.

Tiagabine

Brand Name: Gabitril®.

Dosage Forms: Tablets 2 mg, 4 mg, 12 mg, 16 mg.

Dosage

Starting Dose

Adults and adolescents 12–18 years of age who are already taking enzyme-inducing AEDs: 4 mg twice daily for 1 week.

Children 2–11 years: 0.1 mg/kg/day for 2 weeks.

Titration and Maintenance Dose

Adults who are already taking enzyme-inducing AEDs: After 1 week, increase by 4–8 mg/day at weekly intervals until clinical response is achieved, or up to 56 mg per day. The usual adult maintenance dose is 24–56 mg/day in 2–4 divided doses. If tiagabine is used in a patient who is not taking an enzyme-inducing AED (e.g., patients receiving valproate monotherapy), lower doses (12–22 mg/day) or a slower dose titration schedules are used.

Adolescents 12–18 years of age who are already taking enzyme-inducing AEDs: Increase by 4 mg at the beginning of week two. Thereafter, may increase by 4–8 mg/day at weekly intervals. The daily dosage should be given in 2–4 divided doses. Doses > 32 mg/day have been tolerated rarely.

Children 2–11 years: Increase every 2 weeks by 0.1 mg/kg/day up to a target dosage of 0.4–0.6 mg/kg/day in patients not currently taking enzyme-inducing AEDs. In children taking at least one concomitant enzyme-inducing AED, upward titration may occur every 1–2 weeks, with a higher target dosage of 0.7–1 mg/kg/day.

Note: Dosage adjustment of tiagabine should be considered whenever a change in patient's enzyme-inducing status occurs as a result of the addition, discontinuation, or dose change of the enzyme-inducing agent.

Note: Loading dose is not necessary.

Maximum Dosage Limits

Adults and elderly: 56 mg/day, dependent on concomitant drug therapy.

Adolescents 12–18 years of age: 32 mg/day, dependent on concomitant drug therapy.

Children 2–11 years: 0.6–1 mg/kg/day, dependent on concomitant drug therapy.

Discontinuation Schedule: A dosage reduction of 20%–25% per 2 weeks is safe at the time of discontinuation.

Administration Guidelines

Tiagabine should be taken with food.

Contraindication

Hypersensitivity to tiagabine

Patient Education

1. If you miss a dose, take it as soon as you can. If it is almost time for your next dose, take only that dose. Do not take double or extra doses.
2. Side effects that you should report to your physician as soon as possible include
   confusion
   depression
   difficulty remembering things
   difficulty speaking
   difficulty with movements or with walking
   tingling of the hands or feet
   seizures, whether new or a change in previous seizure pattern
   redness, blistering, peeling or loosening of the skin, including inside the mouth
   skin rash or itching
   sore throat or pain on swallowing
   vomiting
   weakness
3. You may get drowsy or dizzy when you first start taking this medicine. Do not drive, use machinery, or do anything that requires mental alertness until you know how tiagabine affects you. To reduce dizzy or fainting spells, do not sit or stand up quickly. Alcohol can increase drowsiness and dizziness. Avoid alcoholic drinks.
4. If you are going to have surgery, tell your physician that you are taking tiagabine.

See Box 2.27.

Topiramate

Brand Name: Topamax®.

Dosage Forms: Tablets 25 mg, 50 mg 100 mg, 200 mg; capsule, sprinkle 15 mg, 25 mg.

Dosage

Starting Dose for Initial Monotherapy: *Adults, adolescents, and children >10 years:* 25 mg nightly for 1 week.

Children 2–10 years of age: 0.5–1 mg/kg/day for 1–2 weeks.

Titration and Maintenance Dose

Adults, adolescents, and children >10 years: During weeks 2–4 increase gradually (weekly) by 25 mg/day, administered in two daily divided doses, up to 100 mg daily. Initial maintenance dose is 50 mg twice daily. If further increases are needed, increase the daily dose in 50 mg increments on a weekly basis, and dose twice daily. If urgent seizure control is needed, more rapid titration of drug can be performed, starting at 50 mg twice daily.

Children 2–10 years of age: Increase gradually by 0.5–1 mg/kg/day every 1–2 weeks. Recommended maintenance dose is 3–6 mg/kg/day.

Starting Dose for Adjunctive Therapy

Adults and adolescents >17 years: 25 mg/day for 1 week.

Children and adolescents 2–16 years: 1–3 mg/kg/day (maximum initial dose 25 mg/day) for 1 week.

Titration and Maintenance Dose

Adults and adolescents >17 years: Gradually increase by 25 mg weekly until 100 mg total daily dose is reached, administering the drug in two daily divided doses. The recommended initial target dose is 150–200 mg/day administered in 2 divided doses. Higher doses may be used, but doses greater than 400 mg/day rarely will improve responses. Daily doses above 1600 mg have not been studied. *Children and adolescents 2–16 years:* The dose may be increased every 1–2 weeks by increments of no more than 1–3 mg/kg/day. The recommended final daily dose is approximately 5–9 mg/kg/day administered in two divided doses. Dose must be individualized. In clinical trials of patients with Lennox-Gastaut syndrome, doses of topiramate up to 1000 mg/day (approximately 18 mg/kg/day) are used for adjunctive treatment.

Infants and children <2 years: Doses up to 7.7 mg/kg/day, in divided doses, was efficacious and well tolerated. Further study is needed.

Note: For the adjunctive treatment of refractory infantile spasms associated with West syndrome in children, use an initial dosage of 25 mg once daily adding to current anti-epileptic drug regimens. Dosage is increased by 25 mg every 2–3 days until spasms are controlled, or a maximum dosage of 24 mg/kg/day PO given in divided doses is achieved. Over half of the treated children may achieve monotherapy with topiramate after slow reduction of their other AEDs.

Note: It is not necessary to monitor plasma concentrations of topiramate to optimize therapy.

Note: Loading dose is not studied.

Maximum Dosage Limits

Adolescents >16 years, adults, and elderly: More than 600 mg/day is rarely needed, may increase up to 1600 mg/day.

Adolescents <16 years: 9 mg/kg/day for partial or generalized seizures; up to 18 mg/kg/day for Lennox-Gastaut syndrome.

Children >2 years: 9 mg/kg/day for partial or generalized seizures; up to 18 mg/kg/day for Lennox-Gastaut syndrome; higher dosages have occasionally been used in refractory seizure types.

Children <2 years: Safe and effective dose is not established. However, experts administer it to their patients whenever the benefits outweigh the risks. Further studies are recommended.

Discontinuation Schedule: A dosage reduction of 20%–25% per 2 weeks is safe at the time of discontinuation.

Administration Guidelines

Topiramate may be given orally without regard to meals.

Because of the bitter taste, the tablets should not be broken.

The contents of the capsules may be sprinkled on a small amount of soft food (e.g., applesauce, ice cream, or yogurt) for administration. Prepare entire dose and swallow immediately after preparation. Do not chew. Drink fluids to ensure entire dose is swallowed. Do not store any sprinkle/food mixture for use at a later time. Alternatively, you may swallow the whole capsule.

Relative Contraindications

- Hypersensitivity to topiramate
- Metabolic acidosis

Patient Education

1. If you miss a dose, take it as soon as you can. If it is almost time for your next dose, take only that dose. Do not take double or extra doses.
2. Side effects that you should report to your physician as soon as possible include

    agitation, restlessness, irritability, depression, or other changes in mood

    difficulty speaking

    tingling, pain, or numbness in the hands or feet

    difficulty walking or controlling muscle movements

    decreased sweating and/or rise in body temperature

    difficulty breathing; fast or irregular breathing patterns

    eye pain, redness, or swelling

    vision problems, like blurred vision

    hearing impairment

    kidney stones (severe pain in the side or back or on urination)

    nosebleeds

    redness, blistering, peeling or loosening of the skin, including inside the mouth

    skin rash, itching

    stomach pain with nausea or vomiting

    swelling of the face, lips, or tongue

    yellowing of the skin or eyes

    unusual weakness or tiredness.
3. You should drink plenty of fluids while taking topiramate. If you have had kidney stones in the past, this will help to reduce your chances of forming kidney stones.
4. You may get drowsy, dizzy, or have blurred vision. Do not drive, use machinery, or do anything that requires mental alertness until you know how topiramate affects you. To reduce dizziness, do not sit or stand up quickly. Alcohol can increase drowsiness and dizziness. Avoid alcoholic drinks.
5. If you take birth control pills, topiramate may reduce their effectiveness at preventing pregnancy. Talk with your physician about the use of other methods of birth control.
6. If you are going to have surgery, tell your physician that you are taking topiramate.

See Box 2.28.

Box 2.28 Topiramate Precautions

- Abrupt discontinuation
- Breastfeeding
- Pregnancy
- Infants and children
- Elderly
- Status epilepticus
- Closed-angle glaucoma and increased intraocular pressure
- Visual disturbances
- Ambient temperature increase
- Chronic obstructive pulmonary disease
- Emphysema

- Biliary cirrhosis
- Hepatic diseases
- Inborn errors of metabolism
- Diarrhea
- Renal diseases
- Renal impairment
- Nephrolithiasis
- Depression
- Suicidal ideation
- Status asthmaticus
- Surgery

See Chapters 9–14, 18, 22, and 27.

Valproic Acid, Divalproex Sodium

Brand Names: Depacon®, Depakene®, Depakote®, Depakote®-ER, Depakote® Sprinkle.

Dosage Forms

- **Valproic acid (Depakene®):** Capsules 250 mg; syrup 250 mg/5 mL as sodium salt.
- **Divalproex (Depakote®):** Tablets 125 mg, 250 mg, and 500 mg (enteric coated delayed release tablets); extended release tablets 250 mg, 500 mg; capsules 125 mg (Sprinkle). This is a dimer of valproic acid:sodium valproate (1:1).
- **Valproate sodium (Depacon®)**: 500 mg/5 mL.

Dosage

Starting Dose

Adults and children ≥2 years: 7–10 mg/kg/day PO, 3–4 times daily for non-enteric-coated capsules or syrup, twice daily is recommended for delayed-release tablets and once daily for the extended release preparation. A typical adult starting dose is 500 mg daily.

Children <2 years: Not recommended. This population is more at risk for fatal hepatotoxicity from valproic acid.

Titration and Maintenance Dose

Adults and children >10 years: Increase by 5 mg/kg/day at weekly intervals as tolerated and necessary. For most patients not taking enzyme-inducing drugs, optimal clinical response is achieved at doses below 15–20 mg/ kg/day. For patients who do not respond, measure plasma concentrations to determine whether they are within the usual accepted range (50–100 μg/mL).

Children 2–9 years: Younger children, especially those receiving concomitant enzyme-inducing AEDs, may need larger (sometimes >100 mg/kg/ day) maintenance doses to attain target total and unbound serum valproic acid concentrations compared to adults. The extended-release valproic acid is difficult to titrate, and the immediate-release product may be a better choice in young children.

Note: For elderly, use reduced initial dosage and slower dose titration. Dose reductions or discontinuation should be considered in elderly patients with decreased food or fluid intake and in patients with excessive somnolence.

Note: When converting to valproic acid monotherapy from other AEDs, the dosage of the concomitant AED can usually be reduced by 25% every 2 weeks. This reduction can begin at the initiation of valproic acid therapy, or delayed for 1–2 weeks to avoid rebound seizures.

Note: When converting from divalproex delayed-release tablets (Depakote®) to divalproex extended-release tablets (Depakote®-ER), the dosage of Depakote®-ER should be given once daily at a dose 8%–20% higher than the total daily dose of Depakote®. Based on strength, if the Depakote® dose cannot be directly converted to Depakote®-ER, consider increasing the Depakote® total daily dose to the next higher dosage before converting to a daily dose of Depakote®-ER.

Starting dose for the initiation of intravenous treatment in patients unable to tolerate or receive oral therapy
Adults and children >2 years: Initially, 10–15 mg/kg/day IV at 20 mg/min.

Note: For conversion to intravenous dosing in patients, who are currently receiving oral valproic acid therapy from an established dosage regimen, give the normal oral daily dosage by the IV route in an equivalent daily dosage in divided doses every 6 hours.

Note: Patients should be switched from IV to oral products as soon as possible. The use of intravenous administration has not been studied in periods longer than 14 days.

For the treatment of refractory status epilepticus:

Rectal dosage (valproic acid):
Adults: 400–600 mg PR either as an enema or in a wax base suppository.
Children: 20 mg/kg/dose PR.

Intravenous route: Initial loading dose of 20 mg/kg at 20 mg/min, followed by 1 mg/kg/hour with close monitoring; or alternatively, 30 mg/kg at 50 mg/min, followed by 10 mg/kg q6h.

Maximum Dosage Limits
Children >10 years, adults, and elderly: 60 mg/kg/day PO or IV or 3000 mg/day. *Children 2–9 years:* Maximum dosages are not well established; use of Depakote®-ER not recommended.

Children <2 years: Use is not recommended.

Discontinuation Schedule: A dosage reduction of 25% per week is safe at the time of discontinuation.

Administration Guidelines

Oral Administration

- May be administered with food or with a large amount of water to minimize gastrointestinal irritation. May also split doses to minimize GI upset.
- In order to prevent local irritation to the mouth and throat, capsules should be swallowed whole and not chewed or crushed.
- Do not mix oral solution with carbonated beverages because valproic acid will be liberated and may cause an unpleasant taste as well as local irritation to the mouth and throat.
- Sprinkle capsules may be swallowed intact. Alternatively, the capsule contents are sprinkled on a small amount (roughly 5 mL) of semisolid food (e.g., applesauce, pudding) immediately before administration. Do not crush or chew the mixture containing the coated particles. Use any food-drug mixture immediately after preparation; do not store for future use.
- Delayed-release tablets are enteric coated and should be swallowed whole. Do not cut, chew, or crush.
- Extended-release tablets are not bioequivalent to Depakote® delayed-release tablets. Tablets should be swallowed whole. Do not cut, chew, or crush.

Intravenous Administration

- The total daily dose of oral and IV dosages are equivalent. If the total daily dose exceeds 250 mg, the IV dosage should be given in a divided regimen.
- Patients receiving doses near the maximum recommended daily dose of 60 mg/kg/day IV, particularly those not receiving enzyme-inducing drugs, should be monitored more closely.
- Dilute prescribed dose with at least 50 mL of a compatible sterile diluent (D_5W, NS, or lactated Ringer's) for IV administration.
- Administer dosage as an IV infusion over 60 minutes. The recommended infusion rate is generally 20 mg/min.

Rectal Administration

- Valproic acid syrup may be diluted 1:1 with water for use as a retention enema.

Patient Education

1. Swallow valproic acid capsules whole with a drink of water. If valproic acid upsets your stomach, take it with food or milk; do not take it with carbonated drinks.

2. Try not to miss a scheduled dosage. If you take only one dose each day and miss the dose, take it as soon as you remember. If you do not remember until the next day, skip the missed dose and go on with your regular schedule. Do not take double or extra doses. If you take more than one dose a day and miss a dose, take it if you remember within 6 hours. Space the other doses for that day at regular intervals; do not take two doses at once.

3. Side effects that you should report to your physician as soon as possible include

   agitation, restlessness, irritability, or other changes in mood
   blurred or double vision; uncontrollable eye movements
   trembling of hands or arms
   changes in the frequency or severity of seizures
   redness, blistering, peeling or loosening of the skin, including inside the mouth
   skin rash or itching
   stomach pain or cramps
   yellowing of skin or eyes
   unusual bleeding or bruising or pinpoint red spots on the skin
   unusual swelling of the arms or legs
   unusual tiredness or weakness.

4. Do not change brands or dosage forms of valproic acid without discussing the change with your physician.

5. You may get drowsy, dizzy, or have blurred vision. Do not drive, use machinery, or do anything that needs mental alertness until you know how valproic acid affects you. To reduce dizzy or fainting spells, do not sit or stand up quickly. Alcohol can increase drowsiness and dizziness. Avoid alcoholic drinks.

6. Valproic acid can cause blood problems. This can mean slow healing and a risk of infection. Problems can arise if you need dental work and in the day-to-day care of your teeth. Try to avoid damage to your teeth and gums when you brush or floss your teeth.

7. If you are going to have surgery, tell your physician that you are taking valproic acid.

See Box 2.29 and Box 2.30.

Box 2.29 Relative Contraindications to Use of Valproate

- Encephalopathy
- Hepatic diseases
- Pancreatitis

- Urea cycle disorders
- Hypersensitivity to valproate
- Porphyria

See Chapters 13 and 14.

Box 2.30 Valproate Precautions

- Pregnancy
- Breastfeeding
- Neonates
- Infants
- Elderly
- Hypoalbuminemia
- HIV infection/AIDS
- Acute head injury

- Renal diseases
- Coagulopathy
- Thrombocytopenia
- Abrupt discontinuation
- Systemic lupus erythematosus
- Diabetes mellitus

See Chapters 9–13, 16, 18, and 30.

Vigabatrin

Brand Name: Sabril®.

Dosage Forms: Tablet 500 mg.

Dosage:

Adults: 500 mg PO q12h; may increase by 500 mg/day gradually to a maximum of 4 g/day. Lower doses should be used in patients with renal dysfunction.

Children: Doses range from 40–150 mg/kg/day twice a day.

Discontinuation Schedule: A dosage reduction of 500 mg every fifth day is safe at the time of discontinuation.

Patient Education:

1. If you miss a dose of this medicine, take it as soon as possible. However, if it is almost time for your next dose, skip the missed dose and go back to your regular dosing schedule. Do not double the doses.
2. Side effects that you should report to your physician immediately include
   amnesia
   blue-yellow color blindness
   decreased vision or other vision changes
   eye pain
   increase in seizures
   uncontrolled rolling eye movements.
3. If you are taking this medicine for a long time, it is very important that your eye doctor check you approximately every 3 months for any visual problems.
4. You may get drowsy, dizzy, or become less alert. Make sure you know how you react to this medicine before you drive, use machines, or do anything else that could be dangerous if you are dizzy, drowsy, or not alert.

Zonisamide

Brand Name: Zonegran®.

Dosage Forms: Oral capsules 25 mg, 50 mg, and 100 mg.

Dosage

Starting Dose

Adults and adolescents >16 years: 50–100 mg/day, once or twice (divided doses) daily, for 2 weeks.

Adolescents and children <16 years: Safe and effective use has not been established. However, experts suggest an initial dose of 2–4 mg/kg/day once or twice (divided doses) daily.

Titration and Maintenance Dose

Adults and adolescents >16 years: After 2 weeks, the dose may be increased to 200 mg/day once or twice (divided doses) daily for at least 2 weeks. The dose can then be increased to 300 mg once daily and 400 mg once daily every 2 weeks. Usual maintenance dose is 200–400 mg daily. Higher doses are of uncertain benefit. There is little experience with doses greater than 600 mg/day.

Adolescents and children <16 years: Titration is usually slow, with increments of 1–2 mg/kg/day every 1–2 week. The target dosage is 4–8 mg/kg/ day.

Note: Loading dose is not studied.

Maximum Dosage Limits

- *Adolescents >16 years, adults, and elderly:* 600 mg/day.
- *Adolescents <16 years and children:* 12 mg/kg/day.

Discontinuation Schedule: A dosage reduction of 20%–25% per 2 weeks is safe at the time of discontinuation.

Administration Guidelines

Zonisamide may be taken with or without food.

Relative Contraindication

Sulfonamide hypersensitivity

Patient Education

1. Swallow the capsules whole with a drink of water. Do not bite into or break open the capsule.
2. If you miss a dose, take it as soon as you can. If it is almost time for your next dose, take only that dose. Do not take double or extra doses.
3. Side effects that you should report to your physician immediately include

    changes in seizure type or frequency

    decreased sweating or a rise in body temperature

    depression

    seeing or hearing things or people that are not really there unusual thoughts

severe drowsiness, difficulty concentrating, or coordination problems

speech or language problems

difficulty breathing or tightening of the throat

fever, sore throat, sores in your mouth, or easy bruising

redness, blistering, peeling or loosening of the skin, including inside the mouth

skin rash or itching

swelling of lips or tongue

sudden back pain, abdominal pain, pain when urinating, bloody or dark urine

vomiting

4. Drink 6–8 glasses of water a day. This may help to prevent kidney stones.

5. You may get drowsy or dizzy or have coordination problems. Do not drive, use machinery, or do anything that requires mental alertness until you know how zonisamide affects you. To reduce dizzy spells, do not sit or stand up quickly. Alcohol can increase drowsiness and dizziness. Avoid alcoholic drinks or medicines containing alcohol.

6. If you are going to have surgery, tell your physician that you are taking zonisamide.

See Box 2.31.

Box 2.31 Zonisamide Precautions

- Abrupt discontinuation
- Ambient temperature increase
- Dehydration
- Anticholinergic medications
- Pregnancy
- Breastfeeding

- Children
- Hepatic diseases
- Nephrolithiasis
- Renal diseases

See Chapters 9, 10, and 12–14.

References

AHFS Drug Information 2006. American Society of Health System Pharmacists, Bethesda, MD, 2006.

Depacon package insert. Lake Forest, IL: Abbott Laboratories, 2006.

Drug Facts and Comparisons. St. Louis: Wolters Kluwer Health/Facts & Comparisons, 2007.

E-epilepsy. *Information on anti-epilepsy drugs*. Retrieved from http://www.e-epilepsy. org.uk/pages/spc/.

Jarrar RG, Buchhalter JR. Therapeutics in pediatric epilepsy, part 1: the new antiepileptic drugs and the ketogenic diet. *Mayo Clinic Proceedings*, 2003;78:359–370.

Lacy CF, Armstrong LL, Goldman MP, et al. Drug Information Handbook 2007, Lexi-Comp, Hudson, OH.

Mayo Clinic. *Medical information and tools for healthy living*. Retrieved from http://www.mayoclinic.com/health/drug-information.

Osborn HH, Zisfein J, Sparano R. Single-dose oral phenytoin loading. *Annals of Emergency Medicine*. 1987;16: 407–412.

RxList. *Internet drug index for prescription drugs and medications*. Retrieved from http://www.rxlist.com.

Sunovion. http://www.aptiom.com/2014

Eisai. http://www.banzel.com/2014

GSK. http://www.potiga.com/2014

UCB. http://www.vimpat.com/2014

Eisai. http://www.fycompa.com/2014

Lundbeck. http://www.sabril.net/2014

Chapter 3

Mechanisms of Action and Pharmacokinetic Properties of Antiepileptic Drugs

Mechanisms of Action of Antiepileptic Drugs (Levy et al., 2002; Johannessen and Tomson, 2006; *Drug Facts and Comparisons*, 2007; White et al., 2007; Drugs' websites)

At the molecular level, the majority of antiepileptic drugs (AEDs) modulate excitatory and inhibitory neural transmission. Antiepileptic drugs probably exert their anticonvulsant effects both at the cell membrane and intracellularly. The major targets of anticonvulsant drugs include the following:

1. Sodium channels
2. Calcium channels
3. γ-Aminobutyric acid $(GABA)_A$ and $GABA_B$ receptors
4. Potassium channels
5. Glutamate
6. Glutamate receptors including *N*-methyl-D-aspartate (NMDA) receptors, non-NMDA receptors (α-amino-3-hydroxy-5-methylisoxazole [AMPA] and kainic acid [KA] receptors), and metabotropic glutamate receptors
7. Synaptic vesicle proteins

How the various drugs prevent or attenuate seizures is not fully understood, and the mechanisms listed below only summarize some of the known potential effects of these agents on the neurons and glia. In an ideal world, the specific defect(s) would be identified that underlie epilepsy in individual patients, and therapy would then be targeted to correct the dysfunctional mechanism. In reality, identification of the specific defect is rarely possible, and empiric therapy must be planned. There is presently no evidence to support the theoretical concept that use of two or more drugs that possess varying putative mechanisms of action offer clear advantage over use of two or more drugs that share similar putative mechanisms of action. The mechanisms listed below are offered to enhance fundamental understanding of the various agents, so that the reader gains further insight into the drugs.

Acetazolamide

The anticonvulsant activity of acetazolamide may depend on a direct inhibition of carbonic anhydrase in the central nervous system (CNS), which reduces intracellular bicarbonate levels and may thereby reduce depolarizing GABA responses. It also may alter potassium conductance that induces membrane hyperpolarization.

Benzodiazepines

Benzodiazepines exert their effects through enhancement of the GABA-benzodiazepine receptor complex. They bind at the α1, α2, α3, or α5 subunit in combination with a γ subunit of $GABA_A$ receptors. Three types of benzodiazepine (BNZ) receptors are located in the CNS and other tissues. The BNZ_1 receptors are located in the cerebellum and cerebral cortex, the BNZ_2 receptors are located in the cerebral cortex and spinal cord, and the BNZ_3 receptors are located in peripheral tissues. Allosteric (structural) modification of the receptors exerts anticonvulsant activity. Benzodiazepines bind nonspecifically to BNZ_2 receptors (as well as BNZ_1), which ultimately enhance the effects of GABA by increasing GABA affinity for the GABA receptor. Binding of GABA to the site opens the chloride channel, resulting in hyperpolarization of the cell membrane that prevents further excitation of the cell.

Carbamazepine

Carbamazepine blocks use- and voltage-dependent sodium channels, inhibiting sustained repetitive firing of action potentials. Like phenytoin, carbamazepine reduces post-tetanic potentiation of synaptic transmission in the spinal cord. This effect may explain its ability to limit the spread of seizures. At therapeutic concentrations, it may block NMDA receptors as well.

Eslicarbazepine Acetate

The precise mechanism(s) by which eslicarbazepine exerts anticonvulsant activity is unknown, but it probably involves inhibition of voltage-gated sodium channels.

Ethosuximide

Ethosuximide reduces the current in the T-type calcium channel found on primary afferent neurons. Activation of the T-channel causes low-threshold calcium spikes in thalamic relay neurons, which are believed to play a role in the spike-and-wave pattern observed during absence seizures.

Ezogabine

The precise mechanism(s) by which ezogabine exerts anticonvulsant activity is unknown. In vitro studies indicate that ezogabine enhances transmembrane potassium currents mediated by the KCNQ ion channels. By activating KCNQ channels, ezogabine probably stabilizes the resting membrane potential and reduces brain excitability. In vitro studies also suggest that ezogabine may exert therapeutic effects through augmentation of GABA-mediated currents.

Felbamate

Felbamate may be an antagonist at the strychnine-insensitive glycine-recognition site of the NMDA receptor-ionophore complex. Antagonism of the NMDA receptor glycine binding site may block the effects of the excitatory amino acids and suppress seizure activity. Felbamate has also direct interaction with voltage-dependent sodium channels and voltage-sensitive calcium currents and enhances GABA-evoked chloride currents. Felbamate may increase the seizure threshold by attenuating neuronal excitability and may decrease seizure spread.

Gabapentin

Recent studies suggest that gabapentin has a selective inhibitory effect on voltage-gated calcium channels containing the $\alpha 2\delta 1$ subunit, reducing neurotransmitter release from neurons. It may also potentiate ATP-activated inward rectifying potassium channels. In animal studies, gabapentin has increased GABA responses at nonsynaptic sites in neuronal tissues and has reduced the release of monoamine neurotransmitters. In humans, NMR spectroscopy has indicated that gabapentin may increase GABA synthesis.

Lacosamide

The precise mechanism(s) by which lacosamide exerts anticonvulsant activity is unknown. In vitro studies have shown that lacosamide selectively enhances slow inactivation of voltage-gated sodium channels, resulting in stabilization of hyperexcitable neuronal membranes and inhibition of repetitive neuronal firing.

Lamotrigine

Lamotrigine may stabilize neuronal membranes by acting at voltage-sensitive sodium channels. The blocking of sodium channels can decrease the presynaptic release of glutamate and aspartate, resulting in decreased seizure frequency. This mechanism is similar to that of carbamazepine and phenytoin. Lamotrigine is also a weak dihydrofolate reductase inhibitor in vitro and in animal studies. In clinical studies, however, no effect of lamotrigine on folate concentrations has been noted, although it is possible that folate concentrations may decrease during gestation. Lamotrigine has also been found to modulate neurotransmitter release through an interaction with N- and P-type voltage-gated calcium channels.

Levetiracetam

This agent appears to act via the involvement of a novel binding site, the synaptic vesicle protein, SV2A. This protein is involved in exocytosis and neurotransmitter release. Levetiracetam also interferes with release of intracellular Ca^{2+} initiated by Gq-coupled receptor activation.

Oxcarbazepine

The primary antiepileptic activity of oxcarbazepine is attributed to its 10-monohydroxy (MHD) metabolite. Studies indicate that voltage-sensitive sodium channels are blocked, thereby stabilizing neural membranes, inhibiting repetitive neuronal firing, and diminishing synaptic impulse activity.

Modulation of potassium and calcium channels may also be involved. GABA receptors are not affected by oxcarbazepine or MHD with clinical relevance.

Perampanel

The precise mechanism(s) by which perampanel exerts anticonvulsant activity is unknown. Perampanel is a non-competitive antagonist of the ionotropic α-amino-3-hydroxy-5-methyl- 4-isoxazolepropionic acid (AMPA) glutamate receptor on postsynaptic neurons.

Phenobarbital

Phenobarbital and other barbiturates augment GABA responses by promoting the binding of GABA to the receptor and increasing the length of time that chloride channels are open. Phenobarbital also may reduce the effects of glutamate and inhibit neurotransmitter release from nerve terminals, an effect that is mediated by depression of voltage-dependent calcium channels. Phenobarbital inhibits the spread of seizure activity in the cortex, thalamus, and limbic system, and increases the threshold for electrical stimulation of the motor cortex. There is a decrease in both presynaptic and postsynaptic excitability. All actions result in a hyperpolarized cell membrane that prevents further excitation of the cell.

Phenytoin

Phenytoin exerts its anticonvulsant effect mainly by limiting the spread of seizure activity and reducing seizure propagation. Because phenytoin does not elevate the seizure threshold, it is less effective against drug-induced or electroconvulsive-induced seizures. The primary site of action of phenytoin appears to be the motor cortex, where the spread of seizure activity is inhibited. Phenytoin also reduces the maximal activity of brainstem centers responsible for the tonic phase of grand mal seizures. Phenytoin exerts its anticonvulsant effects with less CNS sedation than does phenobarbital. In toxic concentrations, phenytoin is excitatory and can induce seizures.

Mechanisms of Action

1. Major action occurs at therapeutic doses in which drug appears to bind with axonal Na^+ channels in the activated or inactivated state (but not the resting state). Phenytoin prolongs the inactivation state of the Na^+ channel by preventing the opening of the inactivation gate (located in proximity to the cytoplasmic side).
2. Higher doses inhibit Ca^{2+} influx across the cell membrane through voltage-gated Ca^{2+} channels (N-type). The latter effect may explain the ability of phenytoin to inhibit neurotransmitter release of serotonin and norepinephrine.

Pregabalin

Pregabalin is a structural analogue of GABA. Pregabalin is structurally related to gabapentin, but pregabalin has shown greater potency than gabapentin in seizure disorders (3 to 10 times more potent in animal studies). Pregabalin does not show direct GABA-mimetic effects and has no effect on GABAergic mechanisms. Pregabalin reduces neuronal calcium currents by binding to the $\alpha2\delta$ subunit of calcium channels, and this particular mechanism may be responsible for reduced excitatory neurotransmitter release.

Primidone

The anticonvulsant activities of primidone are attributed to both the parent drug and to the active metabolites. Primidone is metabolized to phenobarbital, therefore it shares all the actions of phenobarbital (i.e., raises the seizure threshold and inhibits spread from a seizure focus). Phenylethylmalonamide (PEMA) is the major metabolite of primidone. This is a less potent anticonvulsant than phenobarbital, but it may potentiate the effects of phenobarbital. PEMA is more toxic than primidone.

Rufinamide

The precise mechanism(s) by which rufinamide exerts anticonvulsant activity is unknown. The results of in vitro studies suggest that the main mechanism of action of rufinamide is modulation of the activity of sodium channels and, in particular, prolongation of the inactive state of the channel.

Tiagabine

Tiagabine inhibits neuronal and glial reuptake of GABA by binding to recognition sites associated with the GABA uptake carrier. Tiagabine inhibits the reuptake of GABA, while vigabatrin inhibits enzymatic metabolism of GABA. By blocking GABA reuptake into presynaptic neurons, tiagabine permits more GABA to be available for receptor binding on postsynaptic cells. Unlike tiagabine and vigabatrin, the mechanisms of action of other AEDs indicated for adjunctive treatment of partial seizures are not primarily mediated through GABA transmission.

Topiramate

Topiramate blocks voltage-sensitive sodium channels. Topiramate also enhances the activity of GABA at $GABA_A$ receptors by increasing the frequency at which GABA activates $GABA_A$ receptors. In addition, topiramate inhibits excitatory transmission by antagonizing some types of glutamate receptors. Specifically, topiramate antagonizes the ability of kainate to activate the kainate/AMPA (non-NMDA) subtype of excitatory amino acid (glutamate) receptor. It may also potentiate ATP-activated inward rectifying potassium channels. Topiramate is also a weak carbonic anhydrase inhibitor, which reduces intracellular bicarbonate levels and may thereby reduce depolarizing GABA responses; however, this mechanism is unlikely to contribute to its antiepileptic effects.

Valproate

Valproate has a broad preclinical and clinical profile. Several effects possibly related to mechanisms of action include the following:

- Valproate inhibits Ca^{2+} influx through low threshold T-type channels reducing Ca^{2+} currents, similar to ethosuximide.
- Valproate inhibits sustained high-frequency repetitive firing of neurons by inhibiting Na^+ ion influx through its specific voltage-gated ion channel (similar to phenytoin).

- It is believed that valproate increases brain concentrations of GABA. A number of mechanisms have been proposed, including inhibition of GABA-T action, activation of GABA synthesis via increased GAD activity, and increased release of GABA into the synapse.

Vigabatrin

Vigabatrin potentiates GABA by irreversibly inhibiting GABA-transaminase, the enzyme responsible for degradation of GABA. Anticonvulsant actions appear to be a result of increased GABA concentrations in the midbrain.

Zonisamide

The exact mechanisms of action are unknown. It appears that zonisamide exhibits a dual mechanism of action; it stops the spread of seizures and also suppresses the seizure focus. In vitro pharmacological studies suggest that zonisamide blocks voltage-sensitive sodium channels and reduces voltage-dependent, transient inward currents (T-type calcium currents), thereby stabilizing neuronal membranes and suppressing neuronal hyper-synchronization. Zonisamide also has weak carbonic anhydrase inhibiting activity, but this effect is not thought to be an important contributing factor in the anticonvulsant activity of zonisamide. In animal models, zonisamide has a profile of activity similar to carbamazepine and phenytoin and is more active against the tonic phase than the clonic phase of convulsion.

Pharmacokinetic Properties of Antiepileptic Drugs (Levy et al., 2002; Jarrar and Buchhalter, 2003; Johannessen and Tomson, 2006; *Drug Facts and Comparisons*, 2007; IPCS INCHEM, Drugs' websites)

Acetazolamide

Absorption: Rapid.
Peak serum concentrations: 2–4 hours.
Protein binding: Approximately 90%.
Half-life: 6–9 hours.
Elimination: Renal.

Benzodiazepines

Clonazepam

Absorption: Rapid.
Onset of action: 20–60 minutes.
Duration of action: Up to 6–8 hours in children and up to 12 hours in adults.
Protein binding: Approximately 85%.

Half-life: Approximately 22–33 hours in children and 19–50 hours in adults.
Metabolism: Hepatic.
Elimination: Renal.

Clobazam

Absorption: Rapid.
Peak serum concentrations: 1–4 hours.
Protein binding: Approximately 85%.
Half-life: 11–77 hours.
Metabolism: Hepatic.
Elimination: Renal.

Diazepam

Absorption: Rapid.
Peak serum concentrations (oral dosing): 30 minutes to 2 hours. With the parenteral (IV) or rectal forms, peak blood levels are reached within 15 minutes after administration and are of the same magnitude as after oral administration.
Protein binding: Approximately 98%.
Half-life: 20–50 hours.
Metabolism: Hepatic.
Elimination: Renal.

Lorazepam

Absorption: Rapid.
Peak serum concentrations: 2 hours.
Protein binding: Approximately 90%.
Half-life: 10–20 hours.
Metabolism: Hepatic.
Elimination: Renal.

Nitrazepam

Absorption: Rapid.
Peak serum concentrations: 2 hours.
Protein binding: Approximately 85%–90%.
Half-life: 30 hours.
Metabolism: Hepatic.
Elimination: Renal.

Carbamazepine

Absorption: Slow and variable. The suspension is absorbed faster, and the XR tablets slightly slower, than the conventional tablets.

Peak serum concentrations: 4–5 hours for tablet and 1.5 hours for suspension.
Protein binding: Approximately 76%.
Half-life: 25–65 hours initially and 12–17 hours after repeated dosing (considerably shorter in children).
Metabolism: Hepatic (> 90%). Carbamazepine is a potent hepatic enzyme inducer and can induce its own metabolism. Onset of enzyme induction is at about 3 days, with maximum effect at about 30 days.
Active Metabolite: Carbamazepine 10,11-epoxide.
Elimination: Renal.

Eslicarbazepine Acetate

Absorption: Eslicarbazepine acetate is mostly undetectable after oral administration. Eslicarbazepine, the major metabolite, is primarily responsible for the pharmacological effect of eslicarbazepine acetate. Food has no effect on the pharmacokinetics of eslicarbazepine acetate.
Peak serum concentrations: 1–4 hours.
Protein binding: < 40%.
Half-life: 13–20 hours.
Metabolism: Hepatic. Eslicarbazepine has moderate inhibitory effect on CYP2C19. A mild activation of UGT1A1-mediated glucuronidation was observed in vitro. It can induce CYP3A4.
Active Metabolites: Eslicarbazepine (91%); (R)-licarbazepine 5%; oxcarbazepine 1%.
Elimination: Renal.

Ethosuximide

Absorption: Rapid.
Peak serum concentrations: 4 hours in adults and 3–7 hours in children.
Protein binding: Less than 5%.
Half-life: 60 hours in adults and 30 hours in children.
Metabolism: Hepatic (65%). The hepatic microsomal isoenzyme CYP-3A4 appears to be involved. Ethosuximide does not inhibit or induce the hepatic CYP-450 microsomal enzymes or UDP-glucuronosyltransferase.
Elimination: Renal.

Ezogabine

Absorption: Rapid.
Peak serum concentrations: 0.5–2 hours.
Protein binding: Approximately 22%–30%.
Half-life: 7–11 hours. Coadministration of ezogabine with medications that are inhibitors or inducers of cytochrome P450 enzymes is

unlikely to affect the pharmacokinetics of ezogabine. However, the inducers for uridine 5'-diphosphate (UDP)- glucuronyltransferases (UGTs), such as carbamazepine and phenytoin, may reduce serum levels.
Metabolism: Hepatic.
Elimination: Renal.

Felbamate

Absorption: Rapid.
Peak serum concentrations: 1–6 hours.
Protein binding: Approximately 22%–30%.
Half-life: 14–23 hours in adults; lower in children. The metabolism of felbamate is enhanced by enzyme-inducing AEDs such as phenobarbital, phenytoin, primidone, and carbamazepine, resulting in an average felbamate half-life of approximately 14 hours.
Metabolism: Hepatic (60%).
Elimination: Renal.

Gabapentin

Absorption: Rapid.
Peak serum concentrations: 2–3 hours. In general, the concentration to dose ratio of gabapentin increases significantly with age. Approximately 30% larger doses would be required in younger children (<5 years) to achieve the same exposure as in older children.
Protein binding: Less than 3%.
Half-life: 5–9 hours.
Metabolism: Not metabolized. Gabapentin does not interact with other AEDs to any clinically significant degree.
Elimination: Renal.

Lacosamide

Absorption: Rapid.
Peak serum concentrations: 1–4 hours.
Protein binding: Less than 15%.
Half-life: 13 hours.
Metabolism: Renal.
Elimination: Renal.

Lamotrigine

Absorption: Rapid.
Peak serum concentrations: 1–3 hours. Peak plasma concentrations occur up to 4.8 hours after an oral dose in patients on concomitant

valproic acid. A second peak may be seen 4–6 hours after administration; this may suggest entero-hepatic circulation.

Protein binding: Approximately 55%. It does not displace other AEDs from their protein-binding sites.

Half-life: 14–60 (mean: 24) hours in adults. After multiple dosing in normal adults, lamotrigine may induce its own metabolism, which may decrease the half-life by 25%. Carbamazepine, phenytoin, phenobarbital, and primidone can decrease lamotrigine half-life (to average 15 hours). Valproic acid increases elimination half-life (to average 60 hours), whether given with or without the other AEDs. Clearance in children is up to 2 folds higher than in adults.

Metabolism: Hepatic (> 90%).

Elimination: Renal.

Levetiracetam

Absorption: Rapid.

Peak serum concentrations: 1 hour.

Protein binding: Less than 10%.

Half-life: 5–8 hours.

Metabolism: Not extensively metabolized. Levetiracetam does not interact with other AEDs to any clinically significant degree.

Elimination: Renal.

Oxcarbazepine

Absorption: Rapid.

Peak serum concentrations of MHD: 4–8 hours.

Protein binding: 40% (of MHD).

Half-life: The half-lives of oxcarbazepine and MHD are 2 and 9 hours, respectively. Children 2–6 years have a higher clearance (more than twice) and need a larger dose/kg body weight of oxcarbazepine.

Metabolism: Hepatic. Rapid reduction in the liver to MHD. Mild enzyme inducer.

Elimination: Renal.

Perampanel

Absorption: Rapid.

Peak serum concentrations: 0.5–2.5 hours (fasted condition); 2–3 (fed condition).

Protein binding: About 95%.

Half-life: 105 hours.

Metabolism: Hepatic.

Elimination: Feces and renal.

Phenobarbital

Absorption: Variable.
Onset of action: Onset of action after IV administration is within 5 minutes, reaching a maximum in about 30 minutes. The peak brain/plasma concentration ratio occurs slowly about 20–40 minutes after an IV dose.
Peak serum concentrations: Peak serum concentrations are achieved 8–12 hours after oral dosing.
Protein binding: About 20%–45%.
Half-life: In adults 50–120 hours (mean: 96 hours); in children 37–73 hours (mean: 69 hours); in infants 53–73 hours (mean: 63 hours); in neonates 45–200 hours (mean: 111 hours).
Metabolism: Hepatic (75%). Phenobarbital accelerates the clearance of other drugs metabolized via hepatic microsomal enzymes, but there is no clear evidence that phenobarbital accelerates its own metabolism.
Elimination: Renal.

Phenytoin

Absorption: Variable and slow.
Onset of action: Brain and cerebrospinal fluid concentrations are equal to plasma concentrations 10–20 minutes following an intravenously administered loading dose.
Peak serum concentrations: Rapid-release dosage forms reach peak concentrations in 1.5–6 hours, whereas a dose of sustained-release capsules may not reach peak concentrations for 12 hours. The absorption rate is also dose dependent. Time to achieve peak concentration (T-max) may occur 1–2 hours after a 200-mg oral dose, whereas T-max may not be observed for up to 18 hours after an 800-mg dose. Because the absorption rate of phenytoin is dose dependent, oral loading doses should be administered in divided doses.
Protein binding: About 90%–95%; less in patients with renal failure or hypoproteinemia.
Note: Patients with hepatic failure can have an increase in serum bilirubin concentration, which can displace phenytoin from protein binding sites and increase the free fraction of the drug. Other hypoalbuminemic states with potential for an increased free fraction of phenytoin include major trauma, burns, nephrotic syndrome, malnutrition, or surgery. The measurement of unbound ("free") phenytoin serum concentrations may be helpful in these specific conditions.
Half-life: Because of the saturable metabolism, it is inaccurate to report a fixed value for phenytoin half-life. It depends on dosage and various patient factors. Half-life of the drug is longer when the plasma levels are higher, and plasma levels can rise out of proportion to an increase in dose. The half-life of phenytoin in the low to mid-therapeutic

range varies from 12 to 36 hours (average: 24 hours). For most patients, half-life of 20–60 hours may be found at therapeutic levels.

Note: Fever (≥101 degrees F) for more than 24 hours can also induce hepatic oxidative enzymes and potentially decrease phenytoin serum concentrations. Liver disease can reduce the clearance of phenytoin or, paradoxically, increase its clearance if protein binding is significantly decreased.

Metabolism: Hepatic. Metabolic capacity can be saturated at therapeutic concentrations. Below the saturation point, phenytoin is eliminated in a linear, first-order process. Above the saturation point, elimination is much slower and occurs via a zero-order process. Phenytoin accelerates the clearance of other drugs metabolized via hepatic microsomal enzymes.

Note: Phenytoin dosage forms are available as either phenytoin acid (tablets and oral suspension) or phenytoin sodium (capsules and injection). Phenytoin sodium contains 8% less phenytoin than does phenytoin acid. Due to its unique metabolism, switching patients from phenytoin sodium to phenytoin acid without adjusting the dose to account for this 8% difference could lead to phenytoin toxicity.

Elimination: Renal (metabolites). Less than 5% of phenytoin is eliminated renally.

Pregabalin

Absorption: Rapid.
Peak serum concentrations: 1–1.5 hours.
Protein binding: None.
Half-life: 6 hours.
Metabolism: Negligible (<2%) hepatic metabolism. Pregabalin does not interact with other AEDs to any clinically significant degree.
Elimination: Renal.

Primidone

Absorption: Rapid, but variable.
Peak serum concentrations: 3–4 hours.
Protein binding: Phenylethylmalonamide (PEMA) and primidone are bound only minimally to plasma proteins. About 20%–45% of phenobarbital is plasma protein-bound.
Half-life: Plasma half-life of primidone is 10–12 hours. Plasma half-life of PEMA is 29–36 hours. Both PEMA and phenobarbital, which has a long half-life of several days, accumulate during long-term therapy.
Metabolism: Hepatic. Primidone accelerates the clearance of other drugs metabolized via hepatic microsomal enzymes.
Active metabolites: Phenobarbital and PEMA.
Elimination: Renal.

Rufinamide

Absorption: Slow and dose dependent.
Peak serum concentrations: 4–6 hours.
Protein binding: 34%.
Half-life: 6–10 hours.
Metabolism: Hepatic. The metabolic route is not cytochrome P450 dependent. However, potent cytochrome P450 enzyme inducers, such as carbamazepine and phenytoin increase the clearance of rufinamide and valproate decreases rufinamide clearance. Rufinamide is a weak inhibitor of CYP 2E1 and a weak inducer of CYP 3A4 enzymes.
Elimination: Renal.

Tiagabine

Absorption: Rapid.
Peak serum concentrations: 45 minutes in the fasting state (0.5–2 hours).
Protein binding: 96%. Valproate displaces tiagabine from its binding sites on serum proteins.
Half-life: 4–13 (average: 7) hours. In patients who take hepatic enzyme-inducing drugs, elimination half-life is about 4–7 hours. The mean half-life of tiagabine in children is shorter (3.2 hours in those taking an inducing AED versus 5.7 hours in children taking valproic acid concomitantly).
Metabolism: Hepatic. Tiagabine is thought to be metabolized primarily by the hepatic cytochrome P-450 isoenzyme CYP3A4. Tiagabine does not inhibit or induce the hepatic CYP450 microsomal enzymes.
Elimination: Feces and renal.

Topiramate

Absorption: Rapid.
Peak serum concentrations: 1–4 (average: 2) hours. Children <11 years require much higher doses in mg/kg body weight to achieve drug concentrations comparable to adults.
Protein binding: 13%–41% (average: 15%).
Half-life: 19–25 (mean: 21) hours.
Metabolism: Hepatic (30%).
Elimination: Renal.

Valproate

Absorption: Rapid.
Peak serum concentrations: 1–4 hours following oral administration of the sodium salt or valproic acid and within 3–5 hours for divalproex delayed-release and 4–17 hours following divalproex extended-release tablets.

Protein binding: 90%, but protein binding decreases as the serum concentration increases.
Half-life: 7–20 hours.
Metabolism: Hepatic. Valproic acid inhibits the activity of CYP2C9 and UGT at clinically relevant concentrations in human liver microsomes.
Elimination: Renal.

Vigabatrin

Absorption: Rapid.
Peak serum concentrations: 0.7–1.1 hours.
Protein binding: None.
Half-life: 6–8 hours.
Metabolism: Not metabolized by liver. Vigabatrin does not interact with other AEDs to any clinically significant degree.
Elimination: Renal.

Zonisamide

Absorption: Rapid.
Peak serum concentrations: 2–7 hours.
Protein binding: About 40%–60%. Zonisamide is extensively bound to erythrocytes, resulting in an 8-fold higher concentration of zonisamide in red blood cells than in plasma.
Half-life: In plasma is about 63 hours (50–70 hours) and in red blood cells is approximately 105 hours. The elimination half-life of zonisamide in plasma is about 27–38 hours during combination therapy with enzyme-inducing AEDs.
Metabolism: Hepatic (70%). However, zonisamide does not inhibit or induce cytochrome P-450 enzymes or UGT.
Elimination: Renal.

References

Drug Facts and Comparisons. St. Louis: Wolters Kluwer Health/Facts & Comparisons, 2007.

IPCS INCHEM. *Chemical safety information from intergovernmental organizations.* Retrieved from http://www.inchem.org.

Jarrar RG, Buchhalter JR. Therapeutics in pediatric epilepsy, part 1: the new antiepileptic drugs and the ketogenic diet. *Mayo Clinic Proceedings*. 2003;78: 359–370.

Johannessen SI, Tomson T. Pharmacokinetic variability of newer antiepileptic drugs. *Clinical Pharmacokinetics*. 2006;45: 1061–1075.

Levy RH, Mattson RH, Meldrum BS, Perucca E. *Antiepileptic Drugs*, 5th ed. Philadelphia: Lippincott Williams & Wilkins, 2002.

White HS, Smith MD, Wilcox KS. Mechanisms of action of antiepileptic drugs. *International Review of Neurobiology*. 2007;81: 85–110.

Sunovion. http://www.aptiom.com/2014
Eisai. http://www.banzel.com/2014
GSK. http://www.potiga.com/2014
UCB. http://www.vimpat.com/2014
Eisai. http://www.fycompa.com/2014
Lundbeck. http://www.sabril.net/2014

Chapter 4

Monitoring Antiepileptic Drugs and Their Toxicity

There is a correlation between the serum concentration of any antiepileptic drug (AED) and its therapeutic and toxic effects. Therapeutic drug monitoring seeks to optimize the desirable effects of AEDs, while minimizing their undesirable properties. The role of drug monitoring is somewhat controversial, because the therapeutic level varies from one patient to the next and is not certain for some AEDs. Moreover, it is not clear that higher levels are more effective than lower levels for many agents. Some clinicians hold the view that levels are irrelevant as long as patients are seizure free and do not experience side effects. Ascertaining that seizures are controlled requires hoping that a seizure does not occur while time passes, and this may be unacceptable to many patients. Therefore, there may be advantage to obtaining baseline serum levels to ensure that serum concentrations are within the range generally found in patients who either respond to medication or who take a dose known to be therapeutic.

Indications for drug monitoring of AEDs include (Neels et al., 2004; Johannessen and Tomson, 2006) the following:

1. Newly diagnosed epilepsy to ensure that the drug is in the appropriate target range
2. After change in drug dosage, to assess new drug concentration
3. If there is a lack of clinical response, to assess patient adherence to the drug regimen
4. Presence of mental retardation, to ensure that high levels, often associated with side effects, are not present. These individuals may not be able to voice complaints about adverse effects.
5. Patients with renal or hepatic impairment
6. Pregnant patients, who are subject to significant alterations in levels as pregnancy progresses
7. Patients with poor compliance, to encourage compliance with drug therapy

For AED monitoring, blood samples should be drawn after steady-state concentrations have been achieved, which is at least 5 half-lives after the first dose and once any enzyme induction or inhibition has had an opportunity to take full effect. Sampling in the end-of-dose condition, immediately prior to taking the next dose, provides trough levels that are easily comparable (Neels et al., 2004).

It should be considered that no optimum serum concentration range applies to all patients. Some patients will respond to concentrations below the lower limit of the recommended range, while others will require concentrations above it. In fact, some experts have suggested that the lower limit of the therapeutic range should be disregarded, and any concentration up to the toxic limit should be considered potentially therapeutic. Furthermore, the therapeutic range can be expected to differ in patients on monotherapy compared with those on polytherapy regimens. Thus, drug monitoring is not a substitute for clinical judgment (Johannessen et al., 2003).

In addition to AED serum level monitoring for aforementioned indications, it may be useful to monitor blood or urine parameters such as blood counts, liver enzymes, and others, for adverse effects of AEDs (Leikin and Paloucek, 2002; Johannessen et al., 2003; Neels et al., 2004; Johannessen and Tomson, 2006; *Drug Facts and Comparisons*, 2007; *Thomson PDR*, n.d.). However, the value of regular monitoring of these parameters, although recommended by pharmaceutical manufacturers and government regulatory agencies, has never been proved to be either clinically useful or to enhance safety. Idiosyncratic reactions are neither predictable nor necessarily aborted by medication withdrawal, so periodic monitoring for these effects is unlikely to alter the course of illness; at best, the reaction might be detected sooner. Similarly, many alterations in serum chemistry measures or blood count, such as elevations of liver enzymes in the absence of symptoms, decrease in white blood cell count, or lowering of serum sodium in the absence of symptoms are commonly disregarded by physicians. Detection of these "abnormalities" usually has no consequence or any justifiable consequence. The patients most at risk for serious side effects appear to be those with concurrent illness or preexisting abnormalities in laboratory screening tests.

In view of the above considerations, one might take one of several approaches, each having merit and none with proven advantage.

1. One might take the view that meaningful abnormalities of screening laboratory tests are extraordinarily rare for nearly all drugs and that routine screening is therefore unnecessary and wasteful. Moreover, the value of earlier detection of severe idiosyncratic reaction is uncertain. If only symptomatic abnormalities would result in changing therapy (ignoring asymptomatic abnormalities), then there is no value in assessing patients without symptoms. One would therefore not perform any routine screening and assess only those patients who develop symptoms suggestive of a drug complication.

2. An intermediate approach could be justified. For patients who are to be treated with an AED known to have particular adverse effects (eg, valproate, which rarely causes liver toxicity), one might obtain baseline liver function tests prior to initiating treatment. Should the baseline tests prove normal, then further monitoring is almost certainly unnecessary. Should the baseline tests be abnormal, then periodic monitoring may have some value, because there is evidence that patients with baseline abnormalities are the ones mainly at risk for serious drug reactions.

3. Last, a more active approach might be employed. Routine screening of blood or urine could be performed, adhering to manufacturer recommended guidelines. This approach is tremendously wasteful of medical resources and subjects more than 99% of patients to regular, unnecessary laboratory testing. Its chief justification is that relevant abnormalities might rarely be detected earlier than if routine testing was not done, perhaps avoiding some serious complications. Unfortunately, as noted above, there is no medical evidence that routine screening actually saves lives or prevents drug complications. Therefore, we do not favor this approach.

Acetazolamide

Therapeutic target range (mg/L): 10–15.

Monitoring Parameters
- Intraocular pressure
- Ophthalmologic examination
- Serum bicarbonate (if symptomatic)
- Serum chloride (if symptomatic)

Manifestations and Treatment of Overdose

Manifestations: Lethargy, metabolic acidosis, tachycardia, and tachypnea have been reported and electrolyte imbalances may be expected to occur with acute poisoning. Confusion, lethargy, metabolic acidosis, and bone marrow depression have been reported with chronic toxicity.

Treatment: Decontamination and hemodialysis.

Benzodiazepines

Monitoring Parameters
- CBC (if symptomatic)
- Liver function tests (if symptomatic)

Manifestations and Treatment of Overdose

Manifestations: Somnolence, dysarthria, diplopia, confusion, ataxia, hyperactivity, hypotension, cyanosis, and coma.

Treatment: Decontamination, supportive measures, and flumazenil (the antagonistic action of flumazenil may precipitate seizures in epilepsy patients receiving benzodiazepines).

Carbamazepine

Serum carbamazepine concentrations should be used to guide dosing in all patients. Therapeutic serum concentrations usually range from 4 to 12 µg/mL. Carbamazepine induces its own metabolism. Several weeks of therapy may be required before the appropriate maintenance dose is achieved.

Therapeutic target range (mg/L): 4–12.

Toxic concentrations (mg/L): > 12.

Monitoring Parameters

- CBC (baseline and periodic)
- Serum sodium (if symptomatic)
- Serum carbamazepine concentrations
- EKG (if symptomatic)

Manifestations and Treatment of Overdose

Manifestations: Dizziness, ataxia, cognitive dysfunction, chorea (extrapyramidal), hyperreflexia, mania, encephalopathy, coma, convulsion, myoclonus, tremor, dermatologic reactions, jaundice, ileus, nausea, vomiting, hyperthermia, hyponatremia, atrioventricular block, bradycardia, arrhythmia, hypotension, respiratory depression, blood dyscrasias, and oliguria. Following ingestion of extended-release form of carbamazepine, the first signs and symptoms appear after 1–3 hours. Cardiovascular disorders are generally milder, with severe cardiac complications occurring only when very high doses (> 60 g) have been ingested.

Treatment: Decontamination, supportive therapy, charcoal hemoperfusion, and dialysis in case of renal failure.

Eslicarbazepine Acetate

Therapeutic target range (mg/L): Not well established.

Toxic concentrations (mg/L): Not well established.

Monitoring Parameters

- CBC (if symptomatic)
- Serum sodium and chloride
- Liver function tests
- Thyroid function tests (if symptomatic)

Manifestations and Treatment of Overdose

Manifestations: Hyponatremia, dizziness, nausea, vomiting, somnolence, oral paraesthesia, ataxia, walking difficulties, and diplopia.
Treatment: Decontamination (gastric lavage and/or inactivation by administering activated charcoal), supportive therapy, and hemodialysis.

Ethosuximide

Therapeutic target range (mg/L): 40–100.
Toxic concentrations (mg/L): > 160.

Monitoring Parameters

- CBC (if symptomatic)
- Liver function tests (if symptomatic)

Manifestations and Treatment of Overdose

Manifestations: CNS depression, excessive sedation, coma, ataxia, nausea, vomiting, hypotension, or respiratory depression (slow and shallow).
Treatment: Decontamination, supportive therapy, benzodiazepine for seizure, and hemodialysis.

Ezogabine

Therapeutic target range: Not well established.
Toxic concentrations: Not well established.

Monitoring Parameters

- EKG: QT interval should be monitored in patients taking concomitant medications known to increase the QT interval or with certain heart conditions (e.g., known prolonged QT interval, congestive heart failure, ventricular hypertrophy, hypokalemia, or hypomagnesemia)

Manifestations and Treatment of Overdose

Manifestations: Cardiac arrhythmia, agitation, aggressive behavior, and irritability.
Treatment: Decontamination and supportive therapy.

Felbamate

Therapeutic target range (mg/L): 40–100.
Toxic concentrations (mg/L): Not well established; probably > 120.

Monitoring Parameters

- CBC
- Liver function tests

Note: Full hematologic evaluations should be performed before starting therapy and frequently during therapy. Although it might appear prudent to perform frequent CBCs in patients continuing on felbamate, there is no evidence that such monitoring will allow early detection of marrow suppression before aplastic anemia occurs. Likewise, at present, there is no way to predict who is likely to develop hepatic failure.

Manifestations and Treatment of Overdose

Manifestations: Sedation, reversible downbeat nystagmus, generalized mild motor weakness, ataxia, gastrointestinal upset, and tachycardia.
Treatment: Decontamination and supportive care.

Gabapentin

Therapeutic target range (mg/L): 2–20.
Toxic concentrations: Not well established.

Monitoring Parameters

- WBC (routine monitoring of laboratory parameters rarely necessary)

Manifestations and Treatment of Overdose

Manifestations: Somnolence, fatigue, ataxia, double vision, slurred speech, lethargy, respiratory difficulty, and diarrhea.
Treatment: Decontamination and hemodialysis.

Lacosamide

Therapeutic target range: Not well established. Suggested range 5.0–10.0 µg/mL.
Toxic concentrations: Not established.

Monitoring Parameters

- EKG: In patients with cardiac disease, obtaining an EKG before beginning lacosamide, and after lacosamide is titrated to steady-state, is recommended.

Manifestations and Treatment of Overdose

Manifestations: Usual adverse effects.
Treatment: Decontamination, supportive measures, and possibly hemodialysis.

Lamotrigine

Therapeutic target range (mg/L): 3–15.
Toxic concentrations: Not well established.

Monitoring Parameters

- None

Manifestations and Treatment of Overdose

Manifestations: Ataxia, nystagmus, increased seizures, coma, and intraventricular conduction delay.
Treatment: Decontamination, supportive measures, IV sodium bicarbonate (1–2 mEq/kg) in case of wide-complex tachycardia, and possibly hemodialysis.

Levetiracetam

Therapeutic target range (mg/L): 12–46.
Toxic concentrations: Not well established.

Monitoring Parameters

- None

Manifestations and Treatment of Overdose

Manifestations: Somnolence, agitation, aggression, respiratory depression, and coma.
Treatment: Decontamination, supportive measures, and hemodialysis.

Oxcarbazepine

Therapeutic target range (mg/L): 12–35.
Toxic concentrations: Not well established; probably > 40 mg/L.

Monitoring Parameters

- Serum sodium (mild hyponatremia is common, although symptomatic hyponatremia is uncommon; see Chapter 14).

Manifestations and Treatment of Overdose

Manifestations: Somnolence, ataxia, bradycardia, hypotension, vertigo, tinnitus, and CNS depression.
Treatment: Decontamination and supportive measures.

Perampanel

Therapeutic target range (mg/L): Not well established.
Toxic concentrations: Not well established.

Monitoring Parameters

- None.

Manifestations and Treatment of Overdose

Manifestations: Altered mental status, agitation, and aggressive behavior.
Treatment: Decontamination and supportive measures.

Phenobarbital

Serum phenobarbital concentrations should be used to guide therapy in all patients. Serum concentrations above 10–15 μg/mL are required for control of seizures while serious adverse effects appear when concentrations exceed 35 μg/mL. Minor sedation occurs initially at concentrations of around 5 μg/mL, which is transient. Most references suggest a therapeutic range of 15–40 μg/mL. Plasma levels >50 μg/mL may produce coma or respiratory depression, and levels >80 μg/mL are potentially fatal.

Due to the long half-life of phenobarbital, several weeks of therapy may be required before the appropriate maintenance dose and therapeutic serum concentrations are achieved in the absence of the use of a loading dose.

Therapeutic target range (mg/L): 15–45.
Toxic concentrations (mg/L): > 50.

Monitoring Parameters

- CBC (if symptomatic)
- Liver function tests (if symptomatic)
- Serum phenobarbital concentrations

Manifestations and Treatment of Overdose

> **Manifestations:** Unsteady gait, ataxia, hyporeflexia, asterixis, dysarthria, confusion, change in mental status, myocardial depression, hypothermia, hypotension, pulmonary edema, ptosis, miosis, and extrapyramidal reaction.
>
> **Treatment:** Decontamination, supportive therapy (hypotension and other cardiopulmonary complications), repeated oral doses of activated charcoal, adequate hydration and urinary alkalinization (with IV sodium bicarbonate), and hemodialysis.

Phenytoin

Serum phenytoin concentrations should be used to monitor therapy in all patients receiving phenytoin. Therapeutic serum concentrations are generally considered to be 10–20 µg/mL (equivalent to 1–2 µg/mL unbound or free phenytoin). Free phenytoin levels may be helpful in assessing patients with hypoalbuminemia or with elevated blood urea nitrogen levels. In uremic patients, the free fraction of phenytoin may be more than doubled, leading to serious adverse reactions. It is recommended to quantitate free phenytoin in uremic patients and adjust the dose to maintain the concentration at approximately 2 mg/L (µg/mL). Achieving total serum phenytoin concentrations as high as 30–40 µg/mL may be beneficial in status epilepticus.

Due to variable metabolism and half-life, it may take several days to weeks to reach steady-state serum concentrations at a given maintenance dosage. Determining when to draw serum phenytoin concentrations is patient specific. In emergent or noncompliant situations, serum concentrations may be drawn immediately. When evaluating maintenance doses, trough serum concentrations may be drawn 5–7 days after initiating or changing dosage. When evaluating phenytoin serum concentrations, certain patient characteristics such as fever, trauma, or hepatic disease should be considered, as well as the potential for drug or food interactions. There are marked variations among individuals with respect to plasma phenytoin concentrations and when toxicity occurs.

> **Therapeutic target range (mg/L):** 10–20.
> **Toxic concentrations (mg/L):** >30.
>
> *Monitoring Parameters*
>
> - CBC (if symptomatic)
> - Liver function tests (if symptomatic)
> - Serum phenytoin concentrations

Manifestations and Treatment of Overdose

> **Manifestations:** Manifestations of toxicity are dose dependent (Table 4.1).

Table 4.1 Manifestations of Phenytoin Toxicity Based on Serum Levels

Level	Manifestation
20 µg/mL	Far-lateral nystagmus
30 µg/mL	Ataxia
40 µg/mL	Change in mental status
50 µg/mL	Coma
95 µg/mL	Death (respiratory and circulatory depression)

Treatment: Decontamination and supportive therapy (diuresis and hemodialysis are of little value).

Pregabalin

Therapeutic target range (mg/L): Not well established; probably 2.8–10.

Toxic concentrations: Not well established.

Monitoring Parameters

- Serum creatinine (rarely needed)
- Creatine kinase in patients with muscle pain, weakness, or tenderness

Manifestations and Treatment of Overdose

Manifestations: Somnolence, confusion, agitation, and restlessness.

Treatment: General supportive measures and hemodialysis if necessary.

Note: In overdoses up to 15 grams, no unexpected adverse reactions were reported.

Primidone

Serum concentrations of both primidone and phenobarbital should be monitored in patients receiving primidone. Serum levels correlate well with clinical response. Recommended serum concentration of primidone is 8–12 µg/mL, and for phenobarbital, 15–40 µg/mL. Several weeks of therapy may be required before the appropriate maintenance dose and therapeutic serum concentrations are achieved. Symptoms and treatment of overdose are similar to those for phenobarbital.

Therapeutic target range (mg/L): 8–12.

Toxic concentrations (mg/L): > 15.

Monitoring Parameters

- CBC (if symptomatic)
- Liver function tests (if symptomatic)

Rufinamide

Therapeutic target range (μg/L): Not well established.
Toxic concentrations: Not well established.

Monitoring Parameters

- EKG: Rufinamide is contraindicated in patients with Familial Short QT syndrome. Caution should be used when administering rufinamide with other drugs that shorten the QT interval.

Manifestations and Treatment of Overdose

Manifestations: Usual adverse effects.
Treatment: Decontamination, supportive measures, and possibly hemodialysis.

Tiagabine

Therapeutic target range (μg/L): Not well established; probably 10–235.
Toxic concentrations: Not well established.

Monitoring Parameters

- Liver function tests (rarely needed)

Manifestations and Treatment of Overdose

Manifestations: Dizziness, CNS depression, agitation, ataxia, tremor, weakness, and myoclonus.

Treatment: Decontamination, multiple doses of activated charcoal, and supportive measures.

Topiramate

Therapeutic target range (mg/L): 5–25.
Toxic concentrations: Not well established.

Monitoring Parameters

- Serum bicarbonate (baseline and periodic; in children; see Chapter 14)
- Serum creatinine/blood urea nitrogen (if symptomatic)

Manifestations and Management of Overdose

> **Manifestations:** Acute neurological symptoms, abdominal pain, blurred vision, hypotension, metabolic acidosis, and stupor.
> **Treatment:** Decontamination and hemodialysis.

Valproate

As with all AEDs, dosage should be individualized and adjusted to patient response and adverse effects. Therapeutic valproic acid serum concentrations for epilepsy are generally recommended to be between 50 and 100 µg/mL, although some patients may require higher serum concentrations for proper seizure control. Toxicity may be seen with concentrations exceeding 100–125 µg/mL; however, it is usually seen with concentrations above 200 µg/mL.

> **Therapeutic target range (mg/L):** 50–100.
> **Toxic concentrations (mg/L):** >200.
> *Monitoring Parameters*
> - CBC (if symptomatic)
> - Liver function tests (if symptomatic)
> - Serum ammonia (if symptomatic encephalopathy is present)
> - Serum valproic acid concentrations

Manifestations and Treatment of Overdose

> **Manifestations:** Somnolence, jaundice, acidosis, heart block, and deep coma.
> **Treatment:** Decontamination, supportive measures, hemodialysis, naloxone (caution in patients with epilepsy; could reverse anticonvulsant effects), and carnitine (100 mg/kg loading dose, then 250 mg every 8 hours for 4 days).

Vigabatrin

> **Therapeutic target range (mg/L):** 1–36.
> **Toxic concentrations:** Not well established.
> *Monitoring Parameters*
> - CBC (if symptomatic)

Manifestations and Treatment of Overdose

> **Manifestations:** Mood or mental status changes and delirium.
> **Treatment:** Decontamination, supportive care, and hemodialysis.

Zonisamide

Therapeutic target range (mg/L): Not well established; probably 10–38.

Toxic concentrations (mg/L): > 80.

Monitoring Parameters

- CBC (if symptomatic)
- Liver function tests (if symptomatic)

Manifestations and Treatment of Overdose

Manifestations: Confusion, loss of consciousness, difficult or labored breathing, faintness, slow or irregular heartbeat.

Treatment: Supportive measures. Dialysis may not be effective.

References

Drug Facts and Comparisons. St. Louis: Wolters Kluwer Health/Facts & Comparisons, 2007.

Johannessen SI, Battino D, Berry DJ, Bailer M, Kramer G, Tomson T, Patsalos PN. Therapeutic drug monitoring of the newer antiepileptic drugs. *Therapeutic Drug Monitoring*, 2003;25: 347–363.

Johannessen SI, Tomson T. Pharmacokinetic variability of newer antiepileptic drugs. when is monitoring needed? *Clinical Pharmacokinetics*, 2006;45: 1061–1075.

Leikin JB, Paloucek FP. *Leikin & Paloucek's Poisoning & Toxicology Handbook*, 3rd ed. Hudson, OH: Lexi-Comp Inc., 2002.

Neels HM, Sierens AC, Naelaerts K, Scharpe SL, Hatfield GM, Lambert WE. Therapeutic drug monitoring of old and newer antiepileptic drugs. *Clinical Chemistry and Laboratory Medicine*. 2004;42: 1228–1255.

Thomson PDR: Felbatol. Retrieved from http://www.felbatol.com/pi.pdf.

Sunovion. http://www.aptiom.com/2014

Eisai. http://www.banzel.com/2014

GSK. http://www.potiga.com/2014

UCB. http://www.vimpat.com/2014

Eisai. http://www.fycompa.com/2014

Lundbeck. http://www.sabril.net/2014

Chapter 5

Choices of Antiepileptic Drugs Based on Specific Epilepsy Syndromes and Seizure Types

Variables that affect a specific antiepileptic drug (AED)'s suitability for patients with epilepsy include the following (Glauser et al., 2006):

- **AED-specific variables:** Seizure type or epilepsy syndrome, adverse effects, and drug interactions and formulations (also see Chapter 2 and Chapter 6)
- **Patient-specific variables:** Age, co-medications, and comorbidities (see other chapters)
- **Nation-specific variables:** AED availability and cost. New AEDs are more expensive than old AEDs, and this is an important issue in some patients with limited financial resources.

Box 5.1 describes the various choices of AEDs based on specific epilepsy syndromes or seizure types according to various treatment guidelines and expert opinions.

For many patients, several agents are good choices with regard to efficacy. However, for the generalized epilepsies, valproate may have the greatest efficacy. Valproate has superior efficacy in regard to seizure control in comparison to topiramate, and topiramate is better than lamotrigine. Regarding side effects and tolerability, lamotrigine is better than valproate, and valproate is better than topiramate. With regard to time-to-treatment failure (considering both efficacy and tolerability), valproate is the most effective drug, and lamotrigine is better than topiramate in idiopathic generalized epilepsies (IGE) (Marson et al., 2007). Ethosuximide is efficacious for absences but has no or minimal effect on generalized tonic-clonic seizures (GTCS). Clonazepam is suitable mainly in pure myoclonic epilepsies with no other seizure types, although it may help absences on occasion. Levetiracetam and zonisamide are also effective for IGE, but no data are available that compare them with other agents. Second-line or adjunctive drugs for IGEs include most other AEDs for generalized tonic-clonic seizures and acetazolamide for absence seizures (Panayiotopoulos, 2002). Large, randomized prospective studies are necessary to establish the effectiveness of lacosamide in patients with IGE. In syndromic approach, there is strong evidence-based data to support the use of valproate and ethosuximide for the treatment of childhood absence seizures; valproate, lamotrigine, and levetiracetam are appropriate agents in patients with juvenile myoclonic epilepsy; valproate, topiramate, lamotrigine,

Box 5.1 Choice of Antiepileptic Drug Based on Specific Epilepsy Syndromes or Seizure Types*

Syndrome	Treatment
Neonatal seizures	*Phenobarbital* and phenytoin are commonly used, but more than 50% of patients do not respond to either drug used alone. There are anecdotal reports of nasogastric or oral use of topiramate or levetiracetam in neonates.
Febrile convulsions	Long-term prophylactic therapy after simple febrile seizures is not recommended. Families can be advised to have rectal diazepam available for use as needed. Usually, there is no need for any therapy.
Infantile spasms	*ACTH* is possibly the best treatment. Corticosteroids could be used instead. Vigabatrin is a first-line treatment in patients with tuberous sclerosis, but concerns about retinal toxicity suggest need for serial ophthalmologic screening. Topiramate, lamotrigine, levetiracetam, nitrazepam, pyridoxine, valproate, and zonisamide are also used.
Lennox-Gastaut syndrome	As initial therapy, *valproate* is often a preferred first agent, but lamotrigine and topiramate are also broad-spectrum AEDs with demonstrated efficacy. Lamotrigine may exacerbate myoclonic seizures in some patients. Therapy can begin with topiramate, and low to moderate doses of lamotrigine may then be considered for synergistic action. Clonazepam (for myoclonic seizures), clobazam and levetiracetam are also used. Felbamate is often reasonably effective although it has much greater risk. Steroids may be helpful in idiopathic/cryptogenic cases. Rufinamide is approved for adjunctive treatment of seizures associated with LGS in children 4 years of age and older. It might be preferred to other drugs as a second-line treatment for LGS when drop-attacks are frequent.
Severe myoclonic epilepsy in infancy (Dravet syndrome)	*Valproate*, topiramate, benzodiazepines, phenobarbital, ethosuximide, levetiracetam and melatonin are used with variable benefits. Carbamazepine, phenytoin, vigabatrin, and lamotrigine are probably contraindicated. Stiripentol is an effective and well-tolerated therapy that markedly reduces frequency of prolonged seizures. *Stiripentol currently has Orphan Drug Status classification in the US, but does not have full FDA-approval.*
Epilepsy with myoclonic astatic seizures (Doose syndrome)	*Valproate* is the treatment of choice. Lamotrigine, ethosuximide, benzodiazepines, acetazolamide, levetiracetam, and topiramate are also used. Carbamazepine, phenytoin, and vigabatrin are contraindicated. Rufinamide is a promising therapeutic option.
Symptomatic myoclonic epilepsies	*Valproate* is usually the treatment of choice. Topiramate is also effective. Benzodiazepines, phenobarbital, piracetam, and levetiracetam are also used. Steroids can be used as a last resort in many of the refractory myoclonic epilepsies. Lamotrigine is also effective, but may exacerbate myoclonic seizures.

(continued)

Box 5.1 (Continued)

Syndrome	Treatment
Landau-Kleffner syndrome	As initial therapy, valproic acid or diazepam is often empirically chosen; ethosuximide, sulthiame, and/or other benzodiazepines are used. If this fails, steroids/ACTH is the treatment of choice (with valproate or benzodiazepines). Carbamazepine and possibly phenobarbital and phenytoin have been reported to occasionally exacerbate the syndrome. *Sulthiame is not licensed by the FDA.*
BECTS (Rolandic epilepsy)	In most patients with typical focal idiopathic epilepsy syndromes, medication is not necessary. *Carbamazepine* or oxcarbazepine is commonly used, if necessary. Gabapentin was shown to be efficacious. Valproate, lamotrigine, and levetiracetam are also used.
Benign occipital epilepsies	Valproate or carbamazepine are often the drugs of choice. Clobazam can be used in seizure clusters.
Childhood and juvenile absence epilepsies	*Ethosuximide* (in CAE), *valproate* (in JAE), and lamotrigine are commonly used. Initial choice may be based on perception of tolerability, potential cognitive effects and systemic toxicity, and urgency of need for rapid control. Levetiracetam, topiramate, zonisamide, acetazolamide, and benzodiazepines may also be used.
Juvenile myoclonic epilepsy	*Valproate* is currently the drug of choice. Among newer agents, there is evidence of effectiveness of lamotrigine, levetiracetam, topiramate, and zonisamide. Benzodiazepines are also effective (but may aggravate generalized tonic-clonic seizures).
Children with partial seizures	*Carbamazepine* is considered an acceptable first drug by many, as are *oxcarbazepine, lamotrigine, levetiracetam,* or topiramate, with choice based on tolerability and comorbidities. Zonisamide and valproate may also be used. Phenytoin and phenobarbital are rarely advised as first-line agents.
Adults with partial seizures	*Lamotrigine, levetiracetam, lacosamide,* carbamazepine, oxcarbazepine, eslicarbazepine acetate, phenytoin, topiramate, perampanel, phenobarbital, valproate, gabapentin, tiagabine, pregabalin, and zonisamide may all be used, with choice based on tolerability, comorbidity, coincidental beneficial effects, and cost.
Elderly with partial seizures	*Lamotrigine, levetiracetam,* and carbamazepine are used. Topiramate, valproate, gabapentin, zonisamide, pregabalin, and phenytoin are alternative agents, with choice based on tolerability and comorbidities. Tiagabine and phenobarbital are rarely used.
Children with generalized tonic-clonic (GTC) seizures	Strongest evidence favors *topiramate* among the newer AEDs. Lamotrigine, oxcarbazepine, levetiracetam, zonisamide, valproate, carbamazepine, phenytoin, and phenobarbital are also used. Lamotrigine and felbamate offer benefit for GTC seizures in Lennox-Gastaut syndrome, and many of the others probably do as well in selected patients. Selection may be based on tolerability and comorbidities in the individual patient.

(continued)

Box 5.1 (Continued)

Syndrome	Treatment
Adults with GTC seizures	Valproate, lamotrigine, levetiracetam, lacosamide, topiramate, zonisamide oxcarbazepine, carbamazepine, phenytoin, and phenobarbital are all used, with choice based on tolerability and co-morbidities.
Elderly with GTC seizures	Levetiracetam and lamotrigine are effective, as are nearly all other agents, with choice based on tolerability and comorbidities.
Atonic seizures	Valproate, topiramate, rufinamide, lamotrigine, levetiracetam, felbamate, phenobarbital, and zonisamide are all used, with choice based on tolerability and comorbidities.
Tonic seizures	Valproate, topiramate, rufinamide, lamotrigine, clobazam, levetiracetam, felbamate, phenobarbital, and zonisamide are all used, with choice based on tolerability and comorbidities.

* First-choice drug is given in italics.

From Shorvon (2000), Panayiotopoulos (2002), French et al. (2004), Sankar (2004), Wheless et al. (2005), Glauser et al. (2006), von Stülpnagel et al., 2012, Wirrell et al., 2013, Conry et al., 2014, Coppola et al., 2014.

and levetiracetam are appropriate drugs for patients with primarily generalized tonic-clonic seizures (Beydoun & D'Souza, 2012; Machado et al., 2013). Carbamazepine can be used with caution as an alternative treatment option for refractory IGE, especially in patients in whom the main seizure type is generalized tonic-clonic (Kenyon et al., 2014).

Importantly, some AEDs are generally ill-advised in IGE. These AEDs include phenytoin, carbamazepine, oxcarbazepine, gabapentin, tiagabine, and vigabatrin, and their use is one main cause of pseudo-intractability (Asadi-Pooya et al., 2013). These drugs may aggravate myoclonus (Sazgar & Bourgeois, 2005). Sometimes, carbamazepine may exacerbate absence seizures.

In the localization-related epilepsies, many drugs are potentially good choices with regard to efficacy, and there is probably little difference in this regard. Side-effect profiles, pharmacokinetic properties, and coincidental effects differ among the various drugs, and these often dictate choice of therapy. We favor the use of AEDs that are neither enzyme inducers nor inhibitors and prefer those that have limited interactions with other drugs (e.g., lacosamide, lamotrigine, and levetiracetam). No studies exist that compare all drugs, and few have been conducted that compare several agents. These studies can serve to guide therapeutic choices, but clinicians must use their experience and judgment when prescribing AEDs, because patient populations in the published studies may differ from theirs, and other circumstances may render study conclusions inapplicable. In a comparison study, lamotrigine had the same efficacy as carbamazepine in regard to seizure control for partial seizures, and both drugs were superior to oxcarbazepine, which had similar efficacy as topiramate. Gabapentin had the least efficacy. With respect to side effects and tolerability, lamotrigine was better than gabapentin, gabapentin was better than oxcarbazepine, and oxcarbazepine was better than carbamazepine and topiramate. With regard to time-to-treatment failure (considering both efficacy and tolerability), lamotrigine was the best, oxcarbazepine and carbamazepine were next, and they were better than either topiramate or gabapentin (Marson et al., 2007).

Box 5.2 shows various indications for AEDs in the treatment of patients with epilepsy according to US Food and Drug Administration (FDA) guidelines. These "indications" are based on the studies done by pharmaceutical companies for marketing purposes and do not reflect treatment guidelines according to the expert opinion. Hence, these marketing indications are rather limited and generally do not reflect the full spectrum of efficacy or use. These indications are based upon conclusions drawn from trial data submitted to government regulatory agencies. These agencies typically take a strict view and approve an AED only for the specific circumstance tested. For example, the FDA will only approve a drug for adjunctive therapy if the investigational trial submitted for review has been conducted using that drug only as adjunctive therapy (ie, added on to other drugs). This approach is contrary to medical experience and sensible science. Testing in experimental models does not support the concept that any drug is only effective as an adjunctive agent; every approved agent is efficacious in experimental models when given alone. In addition, human trials may have demonstrated efficacy for indications and conditions not included in official labeling; however, if a pharmaceutical company has not submitted these data to the FDA and requested approval to market the drug for that purpose, then this indication will never be noted in official regulations. Therefore, government-approved indications are often incompatible with clinical practice.

It is noteworthy to mention that generalized convulsive status epilepticus is a medical emergency and should be treated as soon as possible. Urgent control AED treatment following administration of short- acting benzodiazepines is required in all patients who present with status epilepticus (SE), unless the immediate cause is known and corrected (e.g., hypoglycemia). There is conflicting data and differences in expert opinion about which agent is best for urgent control, and the choice often varies based on the particular patient scenario. The preferred agents that are often used for urgent control of SE are intravenous fosphenytoin/phenytoin, valproate sodium, phenobarbital, or levetiracetam. Of these agents, fosphenytoin may be preferred for most patients, with the exception of patients with a history of idiopathic (genetic) generalized epilepsy, where valproate sodium would be the best choice. In patients with known epilepsy who have been on an AED before admission, it is reasonable to provide an IV bolus of this AED, if available, prior to initiating an additional agent (Brophy et al., 2012). Table 5.1 shows the drug dosing of agents commonly used in the management of generalized convulsive status epilepticus.

Box 5.2 Government-Authorized Indications for Marketing of Drugs for Epilepsy

Antiepileptic Drug	FDA-Approved Indications
Acetazolamide	Absence seizures, unlocalized seizures.
Carbamazepine	Partial seizures with complex symptomatology (psychomotor, temporal lobe). Generalized tonic-clonic seizures. Mixed seizure patterns, which include the above, or other partial or generalized seizures. Absence seizures do not appear to be controlled by carbamazepine.
Clonazepam	Alone or as an adjunct in the treatment of Lennox-Gastaut syndrome (petit mal variant), akinetic seizures, and myoclonic seizures. In patients with absence seizures who have failed to respond to succinimides, clonazepam may be useful.
Clobazam	Adjunctive therapy for the treatment of seizures associated with Lennox-Gastaut syndrome.
Eslicarbazepine	Adjunctive treatment of partial-onset seizures.
Ethosuximide	Absence epilepsy.
Ezogabine	Adjunctive treatment of partial-onset seizures in patients aged 18 years and older who have responded inadequately to several alternative treatments and for whom the benefits outweigh the risk of retinal abnormalities and potential decline in visual acuity.
Felbamate	Felbamate is not indicated as a first-line antiepileptic treatment (has serious warnings). Monotherapy or adjunctive therapy in the treatment of partial seizures, with and without generalization in adults with epilepsy and as adjunctive therapy in the treatment of partial and generalized seizures associated with Lennox-Gastaut syndrome in children.
Gabapentin	Adjunctive therapy in the treatment of partial seizures with and without secondary generalization in patients over 12 years of age with epilepsy. Adjunctive therapy in the treatment of partial seizures in pediatric patients aged 3 to 12 years.
Lacosamide	Adjunctive therapy in the treatment of partial-onset seizures in patients with epilepsy aged 17 years and older.
Lamotrigine	Adjunctive therapy for partial seizures, the generalized seizures of Lennox-Gastaut syndrome, and primary generalized tonic-clonic seizures in adults and pediatric patients (≥2 years of age). Conversion to monotherapy in adults with partial seizures who are receiving treatment with carbamazepine, phenytoin, phenobarbital, primidone, or valproate as the single AED.
Levetiracetam	Adjunctive therapy in the treatment of partial onset seizures in adults and children one month of age and older. Adjunctive therapy in the treatment of myoclonic seizures in adults and adolescents 12 years of age and older with juvenile myoclonic epilepsy. Adjunctive therapy in the treatment of primary generalized tonic-clonic seizures in adults and children 6 years of age and older with idiopathic generalized epilepsy.

(continued)

Box 5.2 (Continued)

Antiepileptic Drug	FDA-Approved Indications
Oxcarbazepine	Monotherapy or adjunctive therapy in the treatment of partial seizures in adults and as monotherapy in the treatment of partial seizures in children aged 4 years and older, and as adjunctive therapy in children aged 2 years and older.
Perampanel	Adjunctive therapy for the treatment of partial-onset seizures with or without secondarily generalized seizures in patients with epilepsy aged 12 years and older.
Phenobarbital	Treatment of generalized tonic-clonic and cortical local seizures. Emergency control of certain acute convulsive episodes, such as those associated with status epilepticus, cholera, eclampsia, meningitis, tetanus, and toxic reactions to strychnine or local anesthetics.
Phenytoin	Control of generalized tonic-clonic and complex partial (psychomotor, temporal lobe) seizures and prevention and treatment of seizures occurring during or following neurosurgery.
Pregabalin	Adjunctive therapy in the treatment of partial seizures in adults.
Rufinamide	Adjunctive treatment of seizures associated with Lennox-Gastaut syndrome in children 4 years and older and adults.
Tiagabine	Adjunctive therapy in adults and children 12 years and older in the treatment of partial seizures.
Topiramate	Topiramate is indicated for initial monotherapy in patients 10 years of age and older with partial onset or primary generalized tonic-clonic (GTC) seizures; adjunctive therapy for adults and pediatric patients aged 2 to 16 years with partial onset seizures or primary generalized tonic-clonic seizures; adjunctive therapy for patients 2 years of age and older with seizures associated with Lennox-Gastaut syndrome.
Valproate	Monotherapy and adjunctive therapy in the treatment of patients with complex partial seizures that occur either in isolation or in association with other types of seizures; sole or adjunctive therapy in the treatment of simple and complex absence seizures; adjunct for the treatment of patients with multiple seizure types that include absence seizures.
Vigabatrin	Adjunctive treatment for children 10 years of age and older with refractory complex partial seizures. Babies one month to two years of age with infantile spasms if the possible benefit outweighs the potential risk of vision loss.
Zonisamide	Adjunctive therapy in the treatment of partial seizures in adults with epilepsy.

From Beghi (2004), French et al. (2004), drug websites, and http://www.neurotransmitter.net/epilepsy_drug_reference.html, and http://www.rxlist.com

Table 5.1 Drug dosing of agents commonly used in the management of generalized convulsive status epilepticus

Drug	Initial dosing	Administration rates and alternative dosing recommendations	Serious adverse effects	Considerations
Diazepam	0.15 mg/kg IV up to 10 mg per dose, may repeat in 5 min	Up to 5 mg/min (IVP) Peds: 2–5 years, 0.5 mg/kg (PR); 6–11 years, 0.3 mg/kg (PR); greater than 11 year, 0.2 mg/kg (PR)	Hypotension Respiratory depression	Rapid redistribution (short duration), active metabolite, IV contains propylene glycol
Lorazepam	0.1 mg/kg IV up to 4 mg per dose, may repeat in 5–10 min	Up to 2 mg/min (IVP)	Hypotension Respiratory depression	Dilute 1:1 with saline IV contains propylene glycol
Midazolam	0.2 mg/kg IM up to maximum of 10 mg	Peds: 10 mg IM (>40 kg); 5 mg IM (13–40 kg); 0.2 mg/kg (intranasal); 0.5 mg/kg (buccal)	Respiratory depression Hypotension	Active metabolite, renal elimination, rapid redistribution (short duration)
Fosphenytoin	20 mg PE/kg IV, may give additional 5 mg/kg	Up to 150 mg PE/min; may give additional dose 10 min after loading infusion Peds: up to 3 mg/kg/min	Hypotension Arrhythmias	Compatible in saline, dextrose, and lactated ringers solutions
Lacosamide	200–400 mg IV	200 mg IV over 15 min No pediatric dosing established	PR prolongation Hypotension	Minimal drug interactions Limited experience in treatment of SE

Levetiracetam	1,000–3,000 mg IV Peds: 20–60 mg/kg/ IV	2–5 mg/kg/min IV	Minimal drug interactions Not hepatically metabolized
Phenobarbital	20 mg/kg IV, may give an additional 5–10 mg/kg	50–100 mg/min IV, may give additional dose 10 min after loading infusion	Hypotension Respiratory depression IV contains propylene glycol
Phenytoin	20 mg/kg IV, may give an additional 5–10 mg/kg	Up to 50 mg/min IV; may give additional dose 10 min after loading infusion	Arrhythmias Hypotension Purple glove syndrome Only compatible in saline, IV contains propylene glycol
Topiramate	200–400 mg NG/PO	300–1,600 mg/day orally (divided 2–4 times daily) No pediatric dosing established	Metabolic acidosis No IV formulation available
Valproate Sodium	20–40 mg/kg IV, may give an additional 20 mg/kg	3–6 mg/kg/min, may give additional dose 10 min after loading infusion Peds: 1.5–3 mg/kg/min	Hyperammonemia Pancreatitis Thrombocytopenia Hepatotoxicity Use with caution in patients with traumatic head injury; may be a preferred agent in patients with glioblastoma multiforme

IM intramuscular; *IV* intravenous; *IVP* intravenous push; *min* minute; *NG* nasogastric; *PE* phenytoin equivalents; *Peds* pediatric; *PO* by mouth; *PR* rectal administration.

References

Asadi-Pooya AA, Emami M, Ashjazadeh N, et al. Reasons for uncontrolled seizures in adults: the impact of pseudointractability. *Seizure*. 2013;22(4): 271–274.

Beghi E. Efficacy and tolerability of the new antiepileptic drugs: comparison of two recent guidelines. *Lancet Neurology*. 2004;3: 618–621.

Beydoun A, D'Souza J. Treatment of idiopathic generalized epilepsy—a review of the evidence. *Expert Opin Pharmacother*. 2012;13(9): 1283–1298.

Brophy GM, Bell R, Claassen J, et al. Guidelines for the evaluation and management of status epilepticus. *Neurocrit Care*. 2012;17(1): 3–23.

Conry JA, Ng YT, Kernitsky L, Mitchell WG, Veidemanis R, Drummond R, Isojarvi J, Lee D, Paolicchi JM; OV-1004 Study Investigators. Stable dosages of clobazam for Lennox-Gastaut syndrome are associated with sustained drop-seizure and total-seizure improvements over 3 years. *Epilepsia*. 2014;55(4): 558–567.

Coppola G, Besag F, Cusmai R, et al. Current role of rufinamide in the treatment of childhood epilepsy: literature review and treatment guidelines. *Eur J Paediatr Neurol*. 2014;18(6): 685–690.

Drug reference for FDA approved epilepsy drugs. Retrieved from Epocrates, Inc. http://www.neurotransmitter.net/epilepsy_drug_reference.html/2014.

French JA, Kanner AM, Bautista J, et al. Efficacy and tolerability of the new antiepileptic drugs, II: treatment of refractory epilepsy: report of the Therapeutics and Technology Assessment Subcommittee and Quality Standards Subcommittee of the American Academy of Neurology and the American Epilepsy Society. *Neurology*. 2004;62: 1261–1273.

Glauser T, Ben-Menachem E, Bourgeois B, et al. ILAE treatment guidelines: evidence-based analysis of antiepileptic drug efficacy and effectiveness as initial monotherapy for epileptic seizures and syndromes. *Epilepsia*. 2006;47: 1094–1120.

Kenyon K, Mintzer S, Nei M. Carbamazepine treatment of generalized tonic-clonic seizures in idiopathic generalized epilepsy. *Seizure*. 2014;23(3): 234–236.

Machado RA, García VF, Astencio AG, Cuartas VB. Efficacy and tolerability of lamotrigine in juvenile myoclonic epilepsy in adults: a prospective, unblinded randomized controlled trial. *Seizure*. 2013;22(10): 846–855.

Marson AG, Al-Kharusi AM, Alwaidh M. The SANAD Study of Effectiveness of Carbamazepine, Gabapentin, Lamotrigine, Oxcarbazepine, or Topiramate for Treatment of Partial Epilepsy: an unblinded randomized controlled trial. *Lancet*. 2007;369: 1000–1015.

Marson AG, Al-Kharusi AM, Alwaidh M. The SANAD Study of Effectiveness of Valproate, Lamotrigine, or Topiramate for Generalized and Unclassifiable Epilepsy: an unblinded randomized controlled trial. *Lancet,* 2007;369: 1016–1026.

Panayiotopoulos CP. *A Clinical Guide to Epileptic Syndromes and their Treatment*. Oxford: Bladon Medical Publishing, 2002.

RxList. *The Internet drug index*. Retrieved from RxList Inc. http://www.rxlist.com/2014.

Sankar R. Initial treatment of epilepsy with antiepileptic drugs: pediatric issues. *Neurology*. 2004;63: S30–S39.

Sazgar M, Bourgeois BFD. Aggravation of epilepsy by antiepileptic drugs. *Pediatric Neurology*. 2005;33: 227–234.

Shorvon S. *Handbook of Epilepsy Treatment*. Oxford: Blackwell Science, 2000.

von Stülpnagel C, Coppola G, Striano P, Müller A, Staudt M, Kluger G. First long-term experience with the orphan drug rufinamide in children with myoclonic-astatic epilepsy (Doose syndrome). *Eur J Paediatr Neurol*. 2012;16(5): 459–463.

Wheless JW, Clarke DF, Carpenter D. Treatment of pediatric epilepsy: expert opinion, 2005. *Journal of Child Neurology*. 2005;20(Suppl 11): S1–S56.

Wirrell EC, Laux L, Franz DN, et al. Stiripentol in Dravet syndrome: results of a retrospective U.S. study. *Epilepsia*. 2013;54(9): 1595–1604.

Sunovion. http://www.aptiom.com/2014

Eisai. http://www.banzel.com/2014

GSK. http://www.potiga.com/2014

UCB. http://www.vimpat.com/2014

Eisai. http://www.fycompa.com/2014

Lundbeck. http://www.sabril.net/2014

Chapter 6

Clinically Important Drug Interactions With Antiepileptic Drugs

Drug interactions can occur whenever two or more drugs are administered simultaneously. Most clinically important antiepileptic drug (AED) interactions with other drugs result from induction or inhibition of drug metabolizing hepatic enzymes or significant protein binding properties. However, other mechanisms, including pharmacodynamic interactions, sometimes play a role. Unfortunately, many AEDs are substrates, inducers, or inhibitors of hepatic enzymes and have significant protein binding (Table 6.1). Therefore, drug interactions are common in patients with epilepsy (Patsalos et al., 2002; Anderson et al., 2004; Perucca, 2005; Patsalos 2013). Drug interactions that cause more than a 50% change in drug exposure (area under the plasma drug concentration-versus-time curve [AUC]) or plasma levels usually require dosage adjustments (Bialer, 2005). Typically, cytochrome P-450 enzyme inducers (e.g., carbamazepine, phenytoin, phenobarbital, oxcarbazepine, topiramate) take days to weeks to upregulate the target enzymes; however, enzyme inhibitors (e.g., valproate) have a more immediate effect. Therefore, for example, initiation of as little as 500 mg of valproate per day may necessitate an immediate 50% reduction of the dose of chronically used lamotrigine (Pollard & Delanty, 2007).

Lacosamide, levetiracetam, pregabalin, vigabatrin, and gabapentin do not usually produce clinically significant interactions with other drugs. Patients with renal or hepatic impairment who are taking strong inhibitors of CYP3A4 and CYP2C9 (e.g., valproate) may have a significant increase in exposure to lacosamide. Dose reduction may be necessary in these patients. Eslicarbazepine acetate, ezogabine, lamotrigine, perampanel, rufinamide, tiagabine, topiramate, and zonisamide have moderate drug interactions. Phenobarbital, phenytoin, carbamazepine, primidone, valproate, and felbamate have extensive and important interactions with many drugs.

Clinically Important Interactions Between Antiepileptic Drugs and Other Drugs

Interactions Resulting in Decreased Antiepileptic Drug Plasma Levels

Co-administration of the combined contraceptive pills causes a decrease in serum lamotrigine level by about 50%, which is likely due to the stimulation

Table 6.1 Effects of Antiepileptic Drugs on Hepatic Enzymes and Enzymes Involved in Antiepileptic Drugs Metabolism

Antiepileptic Drug	Effect		
	Induces	**Inhibits**	**Enzymes involved in metabolism**
Acetazolamide	—	CYP3A4	—
Carbamazepine	CYP1A2, CYP2C, CYP3A4, UGTs	—	CYP1A2, CYP2C8, CYP3A4
Clonazepam	—	—	CYP3A4
Eslicarbazepine acetate	CYP3A4	CYP2C19	Esterases, Uridine diphosphate-glucuronosyltransferase
Ethosuximide	—	—	CYP3A4, CYP2B, CYP2E1
Ezogabine	—	—	uridine 5'-diphosphate (UDP)-glucuronyltransferases
Phenobarbital/primidone	CYP1A2, CYP2A6, CYP2B, CYP2C, CYP3A4, UGTs	—	CYP2C9, CYP2C19, CYP2E1
Phenytoin	CYP1A2, CYP2B, CYP2C, CYP3A4, UGTs	—	CYP2C8, CYP2C9, CYP2C19
Valproic acid	—	CYP2C9, UGTs, epoxide hydrolase	CYP2A6, CYP2C9, CYP2C19, UGTs, mitochondrial oxidases
Felbamate	CYP3A4	CYP2C19, β-oxidation	CYP2E1, CYP3A4
Gabapentin	—	—	—
Lacosamide	—	—	CYP3A4, CYP2C9, and CYP2C19
Lamotrigine	UGTs (weak inducer)	—	UGTs
Levetiracetam	—	—	—
Oxcarbazepine	CYP3A4, UGTs	CYP2C19	UGTs
Perampanel	CYP2B6 and CYP3A4/5 and UGTs (weak inducer)	CYP2C8, CYP3A4 and UGTs (weak inhibitor)	CYP3A4 and/or CYP3A5
Pregabalin	—	—	—
Rufinamide	CYP 3A4 (weakly)	CYP 2E1 (weakly)	Carboxylesterases
Tiagabine	—	—	CYP3A4
Topiramate	CYP3A4,* β-oxidation	CYP2C19	Inducible CYP isoforms
Vigabatrin	—	—	—
Zonisamide	—	—	CYP3A4

CYP, cytochrome P-450 isozyme; UGT, UDP glucuronosyltransferase.
*Dose-dependent induction.
From Patsalos et al. (2013) and Anderson (2004).

of uridine glucuronosyltransferase activity by the steroids. This interaction can result in reduced seizure control in some women. Other examples for a clinically important decrease in serum AED concentration due to drug interactions include the marked inhibition of the gastrointestinal absorption of phenytoin, carbamazepine, and phenobarbital given concurrently with antacids; the decrease in serum valproic acid concentration after addition of some antibiotics of the carbapenem class; the decrease in serum phenytoin levels after the addition of ciprofloxacin; the decrease in serum perampanel levels after the addition of rifampin; and decreased serum carbamazepine, perampanel, and phenytoin levels due to increase in their metabolism by St. John's wort (an over-the-counter herb purported as possibly useful in mood stabilization and stress relief) (Novak et al., 2004; Perucca, 2005; Pollard and Delanty, 2007; Patsalos, 2013).

Interactions Resulting in Increased Antiepileptic Drug Plasma Levels

Interactions resulting in elevated serum AED concentrations have been reported mostly with carbamazepine, phenytoin, and phenobarbital. Clarithromycin and erythromycin can increase carbamazepine plasma levels and cause serious adverse effects by inhibiting metabolism of this agent. Similarly, fluoxetine, trazodone, fluconazole, ketoconazole, isoniazid, metronidazole, cimetidine, and verapamil can increase carbamazepine plasma levels. Omeprazole, cimetidine, allopurinol, amiodarone, ketoconazole, fluconazole, isoniazid, sertraline, fluoxetine, fluorouracil, and tamoxifen may increase phenytoin levels by inhibiting its metabolism, and sertraline and antiretroviral protease inhibitors may inhibit lamotrigine metabolism and increase its plasma concentrations (Novak et al., 2004; Perucca, 2005; Pollard and Delanty, 2007). Diltiazem, an inhibitor of CYP3A4, has been reported to increase plasma carbamazepine and phenytoin levels significantly, resulting in toxicity (Novak et al., 2004). Acetazolamide may increase plasma carbamazepine levels by a similar mechanism (Spina et al., 1996). Chloramphenicol may increase plasma phenobarbital levels, and cimetidine, isoniazid, and sertraline may increase plasma valproate levels (Pollard and Delanty, 2007).

Interactions Resulting in Decreased Plasma Levels of Other Drugs

Patients treated with enzyme-inducing AEDs are susceptible to important drug-drug interactions mediated by hepatic microsomal enzyme induction. The list of such interactions is extensive (Table 6.2). Because of practical difficulties in compensating for such interactions, effective use of some of these drugs may not be feasible in enzyme-induced patients (Novak et al., 2004). In some patients (e.g., patients with HIV/AIDS [Mullin et al., 2004; Romanelli et al., 2000] or those requiring anticancer therapy [Oberndorfer et al., 2005; Sperling and Ko, 2006]), the use of AEDs without enzyme-inducing properties is clearly preferred. AEDs that induce metabolism of at least one of the components of contraceptive pills include carbamazepine, eslicarbazepine acetate, felbamate, lamotrigine, oxcarbazepine, perampanel, phenobarbital, phenytoin, primidone, rufinamide, and topiramate (doses >200 mg/day).

Table 6.2 Drugs With Which Hepatic Enzyme Inducer Antiepileptic Drugs Have Clinically Important Interactions

Drug Category	Specific Drugs
Anticoagulant drugs	Dicoumarol, warfarin
Antidepressant drugs	Amitriptyline, amoxapine, bupropion, clomipramine, desipramine, doxepin, imipramine, mianserin, nortriptyline, protriptyline, trimipramine
Antiepileptic drugs	Carbamazepine, ethosuximide, felbamate, lamotrigine, phenytoin, tiagabine, topiramate, valproic acid, zonisamide
Anti-infectious agents	Albendazole, doxycycline, griseofulvin, itraconazole, ketoconazole, mebendazole, metronidazole, voriconazole
Antineoplastic agents	9-Aminocampthotecin, busulfan, cyclophosphamide, etoposide, ifosfamide, irinotecan, methotrexate, nitrosoureas, paclitaxel, procarbazine, tamoxifen, teniposide, thiotepa, topotecan, vinca alkaloids, vincristine
Antipsychotic agents	Chlorpromazine, clozapine, haloperidol, risperidone, quetiapine
Antivirals	Amprenavir, atazanavir, delavirdine, indinavir, nelfinavir, ritonavir, saquinavir, zidovudine
Benzodiazepines	Alprazolam, clonazepam, diazepam, lorazepam, midazolam
Calcium channel blockers	Amlodipine, bepridil, diltiazem, felodipine, isradipine, nisoldipine, nicardipine, nifedipine, nimodipine, nivaldipine, nitrendipine, verapamil
Cardiovascular drugs	Amiodarone, atorvastatin, digoxin, disopyramide, lovastatin, procainamide, propranolol, metoprolol, timolol, quinidine, simvastatin
Corticosteroids	Cortisone, betamethasone, dexamethasone, hydrocortisone, methylprednisolone, prednisolone, prednisone, triamcinolone
Immunosuppressants	Cyclosporine, sirolimus, tacrolimus
Oral contraceptives	Conjugated estrogens, ethinyl estradiol, levonorgestrel, norethindrone
Miscellaneous	Methadone, theophylline

From Spina et al. (1996), Romanelli et al. (2000), Patsalos et al.(2002), Anderson (2004), Mullin et al. (2004), Novak et al. (2004), Bialer (2005), Oberndorfer et al. (2005), Perucca (2005), Sperling and Ko (2006), and Pollard and Delanty (2007).

In patients taking both oral contraceptive pills and one of these AEDs, a double-barrier method or an IUD may be necessary for effective birth control (Pollard and Delanty, 2007).

Interactions Resulting in Increased Plasma Levels of Other Drugs

Valproic acid, due to its enzyme-inhibiting properties, may increase the plasma levels of a variety of drugs, including lorazepam, nimodipine, paroxetine, amitriptyline, nortriptyline, nitrosoureas, and etoposide. For some, such as amitriptyline and nortriptyline, and for some antineoplastic drugs, these interactions may cause toxicity (Perucca, 2005; *Drug Facts and*

Comparisons, 2007). In addition, valproate is a highly protein-bound agent and may displace some drugs (e.g., warfarin) from their binding sites leading to an increased effect (*Drug Facts and Comparisons*, 2007). N-acetyl metabolite of ezogabine inhibited P-glycoprotein—mediated transport of digoxin in a concentration-dependent manner, indicating that this metabolite may inhibit renal clearance of digoxin. Serum levels of digoxin should be monitored when ezogabine is prescribed simultaneously.

Drug Interactions Between AEDs

Most clinically important antiepileptic drug (AED) interactions with other AEDs result from induction or inhibition of drug metabolizing hepatic enzymes. Because often the treatment of epilepsy is lifelong and patients are commonly prescribed polytherapy with other AEDs, interactions are an important consideration in the treatment of epilepsy. For new AEDs, their propensity to interact is particularly important because they are often prescribed as adjunctive polytherapy (Box 6.1) (Patsalos, 2013).

Box 6.1 Metabolic Characteristics of New Antiepileptic Drugs (AEDs) and their Propensity to Interact with Other AEDs		
AED	**Metabolism (hepatic)**	**Propensity to interact metabolically with other AEDs**
		Affects other AEDs / **Affected by other AEDs**
Eslicarbazepine acetate.	Substantial (>99%)	Minimal / Minimal
Felbamate	Moderate (50%)	Minimal / Minimal
Gabapentin	Not metabolized	Non-interacting / Non-interacting
Lacosamide	Moderate (60%; demethylation)	Non-interacting / Minimal
Lamotrigine	Substantial (90%)	Minimal / Moderate
Levetiracetam	Minimal (30%; non-hepatic)	Non-interacting / Minimal
Oxcarbazepine	Substantial (90%)	Minimal / Minimal
Perampanel	Substantial (>98%)	Minimal / Moderate
Pregabalin	Not metabolized	Non-interacting / Non-interacting
Retigabine (ezogabine)	Moderate (70-80%)	Minimal / Minimal
Rufinamide	Substantial (98%)	Minimal / Minimal
Stiripentol	Moderate (75%)	Substantial / Substantial
Tiagabine	Substantial (98%)	Minimal / Minimal
Topiramate	Moderate (50%)	Minimal / Minimal
Vigabatrin	Not metabolized	Non-interacting / Non-interacting
Zonisamide	Moderate (65%)	Minimal / Minimal

Adapted from: Patsalos PN. *Clin Pharmacokinet*. 2013; 52(11): 927–966.

References

Anderson GD. Pharmacogenetics and enzyme induction/inhibition properties of antiepileptic drugs. *Neurology*. 2004;63: S3–S8.

Bialer M. The pharmacokinetics and interactions of new antiepileptic drugs. *Therapeutic Drug Monitoring*. 2005;27: 722–726.

Drug Facts and Comparisons. St. Louis: Wolters Kluwer Health/Facts & Comparisons, 2007.

Mullin P, Green G, Bakshi R. Special populations: the management of seizures in HIV-positive patients. *Current Neurology and Neuroscience Reports*. 2004;4: 308–314.

Novak PH, Ekin-Daukes S, Simpson CR, Milne RM, Helms P, McLay JS. Acute drug prescribing to children on chronic antiepilepsy therapy and the potential for adverse drug interactions in primary care. *British Journal of Clinical Pharmacology*. 2004;59: 712–717.

Oberndorfer S, Piribauer M, Marosi C, Lahrmann H, Hitzenberger P, Grisold W. P-450 enzyme inducing and non-enzyme inducing antiepileptics in glioblastoma patients treated with standard chemotherapy. *Journal of Neurooncology*. 2005;72: 255–260.

Patsalos PN, Froscher W, Pisani F, van Rijn CM. The importance of drug interactions in epilepsy therapy. *Epilepsia*. 2002;43: 365–385.

Patsalos PN. Drug interactions with the newer antiepileptic drugs (AEDs)—part 1: pharmacokinetic and pharmacodynamic interactions between AEDs. *Clin Pharmacokinet*. 2013;52(11): 927–966.

Perucca E. Clinically relevant drug interactions with antiepileptic drugs. *British Journal of Clinical Pharmacology*. 2005;61: 246–255.

Pollard JR, Delanty N. Antiepileptic drug interactions. *Continuum Lifelong Learning Neurology*. 2007;13: 91–105.

Romanelli F, Jennings HR, Nath A, Ryan M, Berger J. Therapeutic dilemma: the use of anticonvulsants in HIV-positive individuals. *Neurology*. 2000;54: 1404–1407.

Sperling MR, Ko J. Seizures and brain tumors. *Seminars in Oncology*, 2006; 33:333–341.

Spina E, Pisani F, Perucca E. Clinically significant pharmacokinetic drug interactions with carbamazepine. *Clinical Pharmacokinetics*. 1996;31: 198–214.

Chapter 7

Aggravation of Seizures by Antiepileptic Drugs

Drugs may sometimes aggravate seizures, defined as an increase in either frequency or severity of existing seizures, emergence of new types of seizures, or the occurrence of status epilepticus. Pharmacodynamic aggravation of epilepsy usually translates into both increased seizure frequency and increased interictal electroencephalographic changes. A doubling or greater in seizure frequency may be considered as evidence for seizure aggravation. Seizure aggravation can occur with virtually all antiepileptic drugs (AEDs) (Somerville, 2002; Gayatri & Livingston, 2006). As the underlying mechanisms for antiseizure effects of AEDs are not fully understood, the mechanisms involved in seizure aggravation cannot be explained with certainty. However, mechanisms underlying AED-induced seizure aggravation may include:

1. Specific drug effects
   - Increased GABA-mediated transmission (vigabatrin, tiagabine, and gabapentin)
   - Blockade of voltage-gated sodium channels (carbamazepine, phenobarbital, phenytoin, and lamotrigine)
2. Secondary loss of efficacy due to tolerance (benzodiazepines)
3. Drug-induced encephalopathy
4. Drug interactions

In any patient with possible seizure aggravation, other potential causes should be considered (e.g., poor compliance, overdosage, acute idiosyncratic side effects, chronic dose-related side effects, intercurrent illness, development or progression of underlying neurological illness) (Genton, 2002; Sazgar & Bourgeois, 2005; Gayatri & Livingston, 2006). Poor adherence/compliance with the medication regimen and intercurrent illness are probably the most common causes of seizure aggravation, and aggravation by AEDs is a diagnosis of exclusion.

AED-induced seizure exacerbation may be observed more frequently in certain epilepsy syndromes of infancy and childhood, specifically if there are multiple seizure types, even if appropriate AEDs are prescribed. These syndromes include Lennox-Gastaut, Landau-Kleffner, myoclonic-astatic epilepsy, severe myoclonic epilepsy of infancy, and electrical status epilepticus of sleep (Sazgar & Bourgeois, 2005). For example, rufinamide (a drug that is developed and approved for treatment of seizures in Lennox-Gastaut syndrome) has a low risk of aggravating seizures in patients with Lennox-Gastaut syndrome (Coppola et al., 2014). Some other patients, including patients with

Table 7.1 Evidence for Antiepileptic Drug–Induced Aggravation of Seizures or Epilepsy Syndromes

Antiepileptic Drug														
Seizure or Syndrome	CBZ	OXC	PHT	LTG	VPA	GBP	VGB	TGB	TPM	BDZ	PB	ETX	LEV	RUF
Absence	3+	1+	3+		1+	1+	2+	1+			1+		1+	
Myoclonias	3+	1+	3+	1+		2+	1+						1+	
GTCS										2+		2+		
JME	2+	1+	2+	1+										
Infantile spasms											1+			
LGS	2+	1+	2+	1+		1+	2+			2+				1+
LKS	1+		1+											
Rolandic	2+			1+	1+									
ESES	2+		2+											
Focal epilepsies	1+			1+	2+	1+	2+	1+	1+				1+	

AED, antiepileptic drug; BDZ, benzodiazepine; CBZ, carbamazepine; ETX, ethosuximide; GBP, gabapentin; LTG, lamotrigine; LEV, levetiracetam; OXC, oxcarbazepine; PB, phenobarbital; PHT, phenytoin; RUF, rufinamide; TGB, tiagabine; TPM, topiramate; VPA, valproic acid; VGB, vigabatrin; GTCS, generalized tonic-clonic seizure; ESES, electrical status epilepticus during sleep; JME, juvenile myoclonic epilepsy; LGS, Lennox-Gastaut syndrome; LKS, Landau-Kleffner syndrome.

Evidence for aggravation: 1+, limited; 2+, moderate; 3+, significant.

From Snead and Hosey (1985), Asconapte et al. (2000), Genton (2002), Sazgar and Bourgeois (2005), Gayatri and Livingston (2006), Thomas et al. (2006), Kothare and Kaleyias (2007), Liu et al. (2012), Coppola et al. (2014).

mental retardation and/or behavioral disorders, may also be more exposed to the risk of pharmacodynamic aggravation of seizures. Therefore, the clinician should choose an AED according to seizure type or, better, to epilepsy syndrome (Genton, 2002). When a definitive diagnosis is not reached in a patient, the use of AEDs with a broad spectrum of activity (e.g., valproate or topiramate) may be less likely to cause seizure exacerbation (Table 7.1).

References

Asconape J, Diedrich A, DellaBadia J. Myoclonus associated with the use of gabapentin. *Epilepsia*. 2000;41: 479–481.

Coppola G, Besag F, Cusmai R, et al. Current role of rufinamide in the treatment of childhood epilepsy: literature review and treatment guidelines. *Eur J Paediatr Neurol*. 2014. pii: S1090-3798(14)00087-7.

Gayatri NA, Livingston JH. Aggravation of epilepsy by anti-epileptic drugs. *Developmental Medicine and Child Neurology*. 2006;48: 394–398.

Genton P. When antiepileptic drugs aggravate epilepsy. *Brain Development*. 2002;22: 75–80.

Kothare SV, Kaleyias J. The adverse effects of antiepileptic drugs in children. *Expert Opinion on Drug Safety*. 2007;6: 251–265.

Liu YH, Wang XL, Deng YC, Zhao G. Levetiracetam-associated aggravation of myoclonic seizure in children. *Seizure*. 2012; 21(10): 807–809.

Sazgar M, Bourgeois BFD. Aggravation of epilepsy by antiepileptic drugs. *Pediatric Neurology*. 2005;33: 227–234.

Snead OC III, Hosey LC. Exacerbation of seizures in children by carbamazepine. *New England Journal of Medicine*. 1985;313: 916–921.

Somerville ER. Aggravation of partial seizures by antiepileptic drugs: is there evidence from clinical trials? *Neurology*. 2002;59; 79–83.

Thomas P, Valton L, Genton P. Absence and myoclonic status epilepticus precipitated by antiepileptic drugs in idiopathic generalized epilepsy. *Brain*. 2006;129: 1281–1292.

Chapter 8

Polytherapy With Antiepileptic Drugs

Most patients with epilepsy require prophylactic antiepileptic drug (AED) therapy. In these patients, a single AED should be started; treatment with a single agent is referred to as *monotherapy*. Choice of the first AED needs to be tailored to the patient and should be based on seizure type or epilepsy syndrome, drug side-effect profile, age and gender of the patient, comorbidities and comedications in the patient, and, finally, cost. Most AEDs should be introduced at low doses with gradual increases in dosage, depending upon the urgency of the situation to establish an effective and tolerable regimen. Drug titration helps minimize concentration-dependent side effects, fosters developing tolerance to sedation or cognitive impairment, and may aid early detection of the emergence of potentially serious adverse reactions (Brodie & Kwan, 2002; Brodie, 2005).

If the first AED produces a significant and intolerable side effect or fails to improve seizure control, an alternative AED should be substituted. The choice of an alternative AED for patients, who have not responded to the first AED, depends primarily on the seizure diagnosis and epilepsy syndrome. Therefore, as a first step, a serious effort should be made to diagnose the seizure type and syndrome (Ben-Menachem, 2014). If the first or second drug is well tolerated, the dose can be increased by increments toward the limit of tolerability aiming for optimal control (Brodie, 2005). However, once two drugs have failed, the chance of seizure freedom with further monotherapy options is very low (Stephen & Brodie, 2002).

Perhaps 60% of newly diagnosed epilepsy patients will have a good response to the above-mentioned strategy and become seizure free on a modest or moderate dose of the first or second choice of AED without developing intolerable side effects. However, about 40% of patients will have "difficult-to-control" epilepsy. Focal epilepsies and symptomatic (structural-metabolic) generalized epilepsies are less likely to be controlled easily than the idiopathic (genetic) generalized epilepsies.

If control is greatly improved but seizure freedom is not achieved by monotherapy, another AED may be added to the first agent. When *polytherapy* (use of more than one AED) should first be tried has not been evaluated by controlled trials, but many physicians advocate combination therapy once two have failed in monotherapy. The second drug may have a different putative mechanism of action or a similar one. There is no good evidence that using two drugs with differing mechanisms of action (i.e., rational polytherapy) is superior to using two drugs with similar mechanisms of action; for example, carbamazepine and phenytoin may interact with the sodium channel at different sites. However, side effects may be worse when drugs with similar mechanisms of action are used, and use of differing drug types may offer benefit with regard to side effects.

How should one add a second drug? The dose of the first drug should often be reduced somewhat when adding a second agent in order to limit the development of side effects. If the first AED combination is not effective or produces untoward side effects, a sequence of combinations could be tried, but seizure freedom will almost certainly not result, and palliation would be the goal of this course of therapy. Triple therapy can be attempted by adding a small dose of a third AED; however, this is to be discouraged. The greater the drug burden, the less likely that polytherapy will be tolerated (Brodie & Kwan, 2002; Stephen & Brodie, 2002; Brodie, 2005), and worsening of seizures can easily result. If polytherapy trials fail to achieve full seizure control, one should revert to the most effective, best-tolerated monotherapy. At the same time, one should consider all possible reasons for uncontrolled seizures, including non-epileptic seizures, pseudointractability (i.e., misclassification and taking the wrong medication for the specific epilepsy syndrome; taking suboptimal doses of an appropriate AED; or poor drug compliance), and medically refractory epilepsy. The mainstay for making a correct diagnosis is having a standardized approach, particularly with regard to taking a detailed clinical history (Asadi-Pooya et al., 2013).

Once adequate trials of two tolerated, appropriately chosen and used AED schedules (whether as monotherapies or in combination) have failed to achieve sustained seizure freedom, other treatment options (e.g., epilepsy surgery) should be considered (Kwan et al., 2010). Additional pharmacotherapy should be used after failure of two AEDs only if epilepsy surgery is not possible or desired by the patient. Vagus nerve stimulation could be considered after failure of three AEDs.

There always should be a balance between efficacy, tolerability, and safety. Polytherapy with AEDs requires several considerations:

1. Knowledge of AEDs' mechanisms of action
2. Spectrum of efficacy of AEDs
3. Knowledge of the side-effect profiles of AEDs
4. Knowledge of drug interactions and pharmacokinetic of AEDs (Brodie & Kwan, 2002; Brodie, 2005)

Based on the above-mentioned considerations, some suggestions are probably useful at the time of making a decision for polytherapy in a patient with difficult-to-control epilepsy (Brodie, 2001; Perucca, 2001; Asconapé, 2002; Patsalos et al., 2002; Stephen & Brodie, 2002; Brodie, 2005; Kwan & Brodie, 2006):

1. Treatment with two AEDs, rarely three AEDs, but not four AEDs may be a useful therapeutic option for patients who do not respond to monotherapy and are not candidates for epilepsy surgery.

2. In patients with difficult-to-control epilepsy or multiple seizure types, AEDs with different mechanisms of action should be considered for the drug regimen since this may have fewer side effects.

3. Broad spectrum drugs such as valproic acid, lamotrigine, topiramate, levetiracetam, and zonisamide may be preferred over those with a more limited clinical efficacy profile such as eslicarbazepine acetate, ezogabine, oxcarbazepine, perampanel, tiagabine, gabapentin, vigabatrin, or pregabalin, particularly in patients with more than one seizure type, depending upon the epilepsy syndrome.

4. Patients with a single seizure type may respond to a pairing which influences an individual ion channel or neurotransmitter system in different ways (e.g., valproate and ethosuximide for absence seizure).

5. Avoid prescribing an AED that may worsen or aggravate the particular seizure type in the patient (e.g., carbamazepine, oxcarbazepine, phenytoin, vigabatrin, and tiagabine may worsen myoclonus and absences) (Refer to Chapter 7).

6. It is advised not to prescribe enzyme-inducing AEDs (phenobarbital, phenytoin, carbamazepine, primidone) with another AED that is a substrate for that particular enzyme system (felbamate, ethosuximide, lamotrigine, oxcarbazepine, perampanel, tiagabine, topiramate, valproate, and zonisamide), or at least consider the clinically important drug interactions.

7. If an enzyme-inhibiting AED (valproate or felbamate) is included in the polytherapy regimen, clinically important drug interactions should be considered (eg, with phenobarbital, carbamazepine, rufinamide, or lamotrigine).

8. It is usually inadvisable to prescribe two AEDs with carbonic anhydrase inhibiting effect (topiramate, zonisamide, and acetazolamide) together.

9. It is usually inadvisable to prescribe two AEDs with significant cognitive side effects together (benzodiazepines, topiramate, phenobarbital, and zonisamide).

10. A pharmacodynamic interaction between carbamazepine (or oxcarbazepine) and lamotrigine may result in neurotoxic reactions (e.g., headache and ataxia). If toxicity occurs, it is advisable to reduce the dose of carbamazepine or oxcarbazepine.

11. Levetiracetam does not have any significant interactions with other AEDs. Even so, pharmacodynamic interactions with carbamazepine have rarely been reported, resulting in carbamazepine toxicity.

12. Lacosamide does not have any significant interactions with other AEDs. The lack of pharmacokinetic interaction does not rule out the possibility of pharmacodynamic interactions, particularly among drugs that might affect the heart conduction system.

13. Gabapentin does not have any significant interactions with other AEDs.

14. Vigabatrin remains drug of last resort because of its propensity to produce visual field defects.

15. Ezogabine and felbamate are often not recommended, because of their propensity to produce retinal pigmentary abnormalities and vision changes, or aplastic anemia and hepatotoxicity, respectively.

16. Some combinations worth considering include:
    a. For *generalized epilepsies:* valproate and lamotrigine; topiramate and lamotrigine; zonisamide and lamotrigine; lamotrigine and clonazepam; valproate and ethosuximide; lamotrigine and ethosuximide; topiramate and ethosuximide; valproate and zonisamide; valproate and levetiracetam; lamotrigine and levetiracetam depending upon seizure type.
    b. For *focal epilepsies:* lacosamide and any other agent; levetiracetam and any other agent; lamotrigine and valproate; topiramate and lamotrigine; carbamazepine, eslicarbazepine acetate, or oxcarbazepine with gabapentin.

References

Asadi-Pooya AA, Emami M, Ashjazadeh N, et al. Reasons for uncontrolled seizures in adults; the impact of pseudointractability. *Seizure.* 2013; 22(4): 271–274.

Asconapé JJ. Some common issues in the use of antiepileptic drugs. *Seminars in Neurology.* 2002;22: 27–39.

Ben-Menachem E. Medical management of refractory epilepsy—practical treatment with novel antiepileptic drugs. *Epilepsia.* 2014;55(Suppl 1): 3–8.

Brodie MJ. Management strategies for refractory localization-related epilepsies. *Epilepsia.* 2001;42(Suppl 3): 27–30.

Brodie MJ. Medical therapy of epilepsy: when to initiate treatment and when to combine? *Journal of Neurology.* 2005;252: 125–130.

Brodie MJ, Kwan P. Staged approach to epilepsy management. *Neurology.* 2002;58: S2–S8.

Kwan P, Brodie MJ. Combination therapy in epilepsy: when and what to use? *Drugs.* 2006;66: 1817–1829.

Kwan P, Arzimanoglou A, Berg AT, et al. Definition of drug resistant epilepsy: consensus proposal by the ad hoc Task Force of the ILAE Commission on Therapeutic Strategies. *Epilepsia.* 2010;51(6): 1069–1077.

Patsalos PN, Froscher W, Pisani F, van Rijn CM. The importance of drug interactions in epilepsy therapy. *Epilepsia.* 2002;43: 365–385.

Perucca E. The management of refractory idiopathic epilepsies. *Epilepsia.* 2001;42(Supp1.3): 31–35.

Stephen LJ, Brodie MJ. Seizure freedom with more than one antiepileptic drug. *Seizure.* 2002;11: 349–351.

Chapter 9

Antiepileptic Drugs in Pregnancy

Due to the potential for teratogenesis and other impairments and problems (e.g., pregnancy loss), the risks and benefits of antiepileptic drug (AED) therapy should be weighed carefully in pregnant women or in women of child-bearing potential. Pregnancy should be planned in a patient receiving AEDs, so that appropriate measures can be taken in advance. The question should be raised whether anticonvulsant medication is still required, which drug is needed, and what dose should be prescribed. Consideration must be given both to maintaining seizure control and minimizing fetal risk.

Regrettably, there is still a lack of adequate data regarding fetal risk for most AEDs, so comparisons of risk often cannot be drawn. What knowledge exists is fragmentary and limited. Many studies report only the results of the examination of newborns, so malformations and problems that first become apparent after the neonatal period are underreported. The long-term effects of most AEDs on child development are largely unknown. Therefore, the true incidence of major congenital malformations (MCMs) and other developmental problems remains uncertain.

Some general statements can be made, however. The risk of major malformation in the offspring of women in the general population is approximately 2%. The risk of major malformation in the offspring of women with epilepsy who take AEDs is approximately doubled or tripled to 4%–6% on average. Women who take multiple AEDs may have a 10%–12% risk of having a baby with a major malformation, so polypharmacy poses significantly greater risk. Likewise, in women with refractory epilepsy and with high serum levels of AEDs, the risk is high (Penovich et al., 2004). Strong evidence now exists that AED total daily dose is an important factor in determining the magnitude of risk for MCMs; the lowest effective dose should thus be established before pregnancy starts, regardless of which AED the woman is taking. (Campbell et al., 2014; Tomson et al., 2015). Various series report different risks for individual AEDs, but some common themes are apparent. For the drugs for which information is available, the risk of valproate appears to be the highest. Of babies born to women taking valproate, 9.3%–9.7% display major malformations, and as many as one-third of children born to women taking valproate during pregnancy have measurable cognitive and learning difficulties (Meador & Zupanc, 2004; Thomas, 2006; Campbell et al., 2014). The propensity for fetal malformation with valproate may be subject to a dose effect, with problems occurring mainly in women taking doses greater than 1000 mg per day. Levetiracetam appears to have a relatively low risk of producing major malformations. Lamotrigine appears to have a relatively low risk of producing major malformations, approximately 2%–2.9%. However, there may be a dose effect (>200 mg/day may have a higher risk). Early data with regard to oxcarbazepine and gabapentin appear promising, but more are needed (Mølgaard-Nielsen & Hviid, 2011). The other newer AEDs still lack sufficient data to draw any conclusions. The older AEDs, such as phenytoin, carbamazepine, pheno-barbital, and primidone, all carry an intermediate risk, perhaps 3%–6%, of producing major malformations, and some may be associated with lower IQ in children born to women taking these agents (Meador & Zupanc, 2004; Weiner & Buhimschi, 2004; Pennel, 2005; Meador et al., 2006; Ornoy, 2006; Thomas, 2006; perinatology.com, n.d.).

Hence, what is one to do? Several principles can be formulated to treat women who plan to become pregnant. First, implement appropriate treatment before pregnancy occurs (ie, pregnancy must be planned). Aim for therapy with a single agent, ideally one with a favorable teratogenic profile, and use the lowest possible dose of that drug. Aim for seizure freedom with that treatment, because seizures may cause injury to the woman and lead to fetal abnormalities. Avoid polypharmacy. Place women who may become pregnant on a multivitamin and folic acid regimen before pregnancy occurs, in hopes of minimizing birth defects. The optimal dose of folate is not known; most practitioners prescribe between 1 mg and 5 mg daily. We recommend 5 mg folate supplementation when the patient takes valproate and 1 mg while taking other AEDs, as high-dose folate might have important drug interactions with some AEDs. Administration of large doses of folic acid can decrease blood levels of phenytoin, phenobarbital, and carbamazepine, potentially interfering with seizure control (Asadi-Pooya et al. 2008; Asadi-Pooya, 2015). Vitamins and folate should be continued throughout the pregnancy. Have women avoid other products known to cause birth defects or problems, such as alcohol, caffeine, tobacco, and other teratogenic drugs (if possible) (Meador & Zupanc, 2004; Penovich et al., 2004; Weiner & Buhimschi, 2004; Pennel, 2005; Meador et al., 2006; Ornoy, 2006; Thomas, 2006; perinatology. com, n.d.).

Because valproate seems at present to be the least desirable AED, switch to another less teratogenic AED prior to pregnancy, *if possible*. However, when the epilepsy is well controlled only with valproate and other AEDs have been proved ineffective, then valproate should be continued, discussing relevant issues with the prospective parents. One should avoid changing to a new medication during pregnancy if possible, especially early in the pregnancy, because the consequences of using multiple drugs may be deleterious. The AED should be given in divided doses, as the effects on the fetus may be dependent on the concentration peaks. In addition, 10 mg of vitamin K should be administered daily starting at the 36th week of pregnancy to the mother, and the newborn should receive 1 mg of vitamin K intramuscularly at birth. This is certainly appropriate for women taking enzyme-inducing drugs; it is not known whether women taking other drugs require this regimen, but it seems sensible to follow it until more is known. The pregnancy of an AED-treated patient has to be considered as a "high-risk" pregnancy, because there is an approximate doubling of the risk of pregnancy complications. This includes first-trimester ultrasonography and α-fetoprotein levels in maternal blood for the diagnosis of neural tube defects, ultrasound during weeks 19–23 of pregnancy to detect major anomalies, and fetal echocardiography to detect congenital cardiac defects (Penovich et al., 2004; Ornoy, 2006; Thomas, 2006).

In most women, AED dosages must be adjusted during pregnancy. Increases in blood volume, renal clearance, hormonal interactions, and changes in hepatic metabolic activity usually lead to reductions in serum levels of AEDs. Therefore, increases in dosage may be necessary to maintain seizure control. Some of the changes in drug levels may occur very early in the pregnancy. Measurement of serum levels prior to pregnancy and during pregnancy may help guide dosage. A caution must be given that seizure control may be independent of serum level during pregnancy in some women. Despite the ambiguities, we advise measuring serum levels every 2 months or so, and this may be done more often if seizures occur. For example, lamotrigine doses may need to be tripled in some women to maintain prepregnancy levels if that is desired. Once the pregnancy has ended, doses can usually begin to be reduced rapidly, using clinical assessment of side effects and therapeutic monitoring to guide adjustment in dosage. For most AEDs, the pharmacokinetics in the mother will return to prepregnancy levels within 10–14 days after delivery. Lamotrigine has been observed to return to prepregnancy kinetics within the first 3 postpartum days (Penovich et al., 2004; Thomas, 2006).

Food and Drug Administration (FDA) Rating for Antiepileptic Drug Use in Pregnancy (Weiner and Buhimschi, 2004; *FDA use-in-pregnancy ratings,* n.d.)

1. **FDA pregnancy risk category D AEDs:** Benzodiazepines, carbamazepine, phenobarbital, phenytoin, primidone, topiramate, and valproic acid.
2. **FDA pregnancy risk category C AEDs:** Acetazolamide, eslicarbazepine acetate, ethosuximide, ezogabine, felbamate, gabapentin, lacosamide, lamotrigine, levetiracetam, oxcarbazepine, perampanel, pregabalin, rufinamide, tiagabine, vigabatrin, and zonisamide.

Category C means either (1) animal studies have shown an adverse effect, and there are no adequate and well-controlled studies in humans or (2) no animal studies have been conducted, and there are no adequate and well-controlled studies in pregnant women. Category D means that either adequate well-controlled or observational studies in pregnant women have demonstrated a risk to the fetus. However, the benefits of therapy may outweigh the potential risk. For example, a drug may be acceptable if needed in a life-threatening situation or serious disease for which safer drugs cannot be used or are ineffective.

Many AEDs appear to cause a similar group of minor anomalies known as the fetal anticonvulsant syndrome. These include craniofacial and digital anomalies, which become less apparent as the child grows. There is also a 1%–6% incidence of major anomalies, including cardiac defects, cleft lip and palate, microcephaly, and developmental delay (*FDA use-in-pregnancy ratings,* n.d.).

Fetal Risk Summary of Antiepileptic Drugs Based on Human Data (Weiner and Buhimschi, 2004; Pennel, 2005; Meador et al., 2006; Ornoy, 2006, Drug's websites)

1. **Acetazolamide:** Data are not available.
2. **Benzodiazepines:** Cardiovascular defects.
3. **Carbamazepine**
   - Neural tube defects
   - Craniofacial defects
   - Cleft palate
   - Cardiovascular malformations
   - Urogenital anomalies
   - Developmental delay
   - Anomalies involving various body systems
4. **Ethosuximide**
   - Cardiovascular malformations
   - Cleft lip/palate
   - Hydrocephalus
   - Mongoloid facies
5. **Felbamate:** Data are not available.
6. **Gabapentin:** Not enough data are available. Ventricular septal defect has been reported (Morrow et al., 2006).
7. **Lamotrigine**
   - Neural tube defects
   - Esophageal malformation
   - Cleft palate
   - Club foot
   - Cardiovascular malformations
8. **Levetiracetam:** Insufficient data; no significant problems found thus far.
9. **Oxcarbazepine:** Data are not available.
10. **Phenobarbital**
    - Cardiovascular malformations
    - Cleft lip/palate
    - Neural tube defects
    - Limb anomalies
    - Urogenital anomalies
    - Neurobehavioral developmental problems

11. **Phenytoin**
    - Central nervous system anomalies
    - Craniofacial defects
    - Limb anomalies
    - Cardiovascular malformations
    - Cleft lip/palate
    - Physical and mental growth impairment
    - Many other anomalies
12. **Pregabalin:** Data are not available.
13. **Tiagabine:** Data are not available.
14. **Topiramate:** Limited data. Cleft lip and palate and hypospadias have been reported.
15. **Valproate**
    - Neural tube defects
    - Cardiovascular malformations
    - Facial defects
    - Cleft lip/palate
    - Urogenital defects
    - Developmental delay
    - Many other anomalies
    - Cognitive impairment, low IQ: in a recent study, it was observed that fetal valproate exposure has dose-dependent associations with reduced cognitive abilities across a range of domains at 6 years of age. Mean IQs were higher in children exposed to periconceptional folate than they were in unexposed children (Meador et al., 2013).
16. **Vigabatrin:** Congenital cardiac defects, congenital external ear anomaly, congenital hemangioma, congenital hydronephrosis, congenital male genital malformation, congenital oral malformation, congenital vesicoureteric reflux, dentofacial anomaly, dysmorphism, fetal anticonvulsant syndrome, hamartomas, hip dysplasia, limb malformation, limb reduction defect, low set ears, renal aplasia, retinitis pigmentosa, and supernumerary nipple have been reported.
17. **Zonisamide:** A variety of fetal abnormalities, including cardiovascular defects, and embryo-fetal deaths occurred with zonisamide.
18. New AEDs (ie, eslicarbazepine acetate, ezogabine, lacosamide, perampanel, and rufinamide): not enough information is available.

References

Asadi-Pooya AA, Mintzer S, Sperling, MR. Nutritional supplements, foods, and epilepsy: is there a relationship? *Epilepsia.* 2008;49(11): 1819–1827.

Asadi-Pooya AA. High dose folic acid supplementation in women with epilepsy: are we sure it is safe? *Seizure.* 2015;27: 51–53.

Campbell E, Kennedy F, Russell A, et al. Malformation risks of antiepileptic drug monotherapies in pregnancy: updated results from the UK and Ireland Epilepsy and Pregnancy Registers. *J Neurol Neurosurg Psychiatry.* 2014;85(9): 1029–1034.

FDA use-in-pregnancy ratings. Retrieved from Focus Information Technology, Inc. http://www.perinatology.com/ exposures/Drugs/FDACategories. htm./2014.

Meador KJ, Baker GA, Finnel RH, et al. In utero antiepileptic drug exposure: fetal death and malformations. *Neurology.* 2006;67: 407–412.

Meador LJ, Zupanc ML. Neurodevelopmental outcomes of children born to mothers with epilepsy. *Cleveland Clinic Journal of Medicine.* 2004;71(Suppl 2): S38–S41.

Meador KJ, Baker GA, Browning N, et al. Fetal antiepileptic drug exposure and cognitive outcomes at age 6 years (NEAD study): a prospective observational study. *Lancet Neurol.* 2013;12(3): 244–252.

Mølgaard-Nielsen D, Hviid A. Newer-generation antiepileptic drugs and the risk of major birth defects. *JAMA.* 2011;305(19): 1996–2002.

Morrow J, Russell A, Guthrie E, et al. Malformations risks of antiepileptic drugs in pregnancy: a prospective study from the UK Epilepsy and Pregnancy Register. *Journal of Neurology, Neurosurgery, and Psychiatry.* 2006;77: 193–198.

Ornoy A. Neuroteratogens in man: an overview with special emphasis on the teratogenicity of antiepileptic drugs in pregnancy. *Reproduction and Toxicology.* 2006;22: 214–226.

Pennel PB. Using current evidence in selecting antiepileptic drugs for use during pregnancy. *Epilepsy Currents.* 2005;5: 45–51.

Penovich PE, Eck K, Economou VV. Recommendations for the care of women with epilepsy. *Cleveland Clinic Journal of Medicine.* 2004;71(Suppl 2): S49–S57.

Thomas SV. Management of epilepsy and pregnancy. *Journal of Postgraduate Medicine.* 2006;52: 57–64.

Tomson T, Xue H, Battino D. Major congenital malformations in children of women with epilepsy. *Seizure.* 2015;28: 46–50.

Weiner CP, Buhimschi C. *Drugs for Pregnant and Lactating Women.* Philadelphia: Churchill Livingstone, 2004.

Lundbeck. http://www.sabril.net/2014

Chapter 10

Antiepileptic Drugs in Lactating Women

Breastfeeding is generally encouraged for a variety of health and psychological reasons. However, the breast milk of women who take antiepileptic drugs (AEDs) contains these drugs, which are delivered to the baby with each feeding. The obvious consequences of AED ingestion in infants include drowsiness and other adverse effects of AEDs. However, some effects may not be readily apparent. There is evidence in animals that brain development is adversely affected in newborn animals subjected to AED treatment after birth. Phenytoin and valproate may cause reduced brain weight and reduced incorporation of amino acids in myelin and nuclear proteins (Patsalos & Wiggins, 1982). Phenytoin may affect the posttranslational phosphorylation of actin and other cytoskeletal proteins, thereby altering dendritic patterns (Ruiz et al., 1987). Other agents, including phenobarbital, may hinder normal dendritic arborization and alter axon development (Bergman et al., 1982; Hall et al., 2002). Little information is available about other agents; the lack of information should *not* be construed as indicating lack of risk. Moreover, some agents, particularly barbiturates, are not easily cleared by neonatal hepatic enzymes and may accumulate in the newborn.

Therefore, breastfeeding raises significant issues when the mother must take an AED. Ideally, the potential benefits of breastfeeding would be weighed against the risks of the drug so a sensible decision can be made. Regrettably, scientific evidence is insufficiently robust to intelligently compare the risks and benefits of breastfeeding when the mother is taking an AED. While the benefits of breastfeeding are established, the magnitude of these benefits is difficult to measure. Similarly, data regarding risks are only definitively established in animals. As a matter of fact, in one recent human study, no adverse effects of AED (ie, carbamazepine, lamotrigine, phenytoin, or valproate) exposure via breast milk were observed at age 6 years. In this study, breastfed children exhibited higher IQ and enhanced verbal abilities. However, the authors recommended that additional studies are needed to fully delineate the effects of all AEDs (Meador et al., 2014). Nonetheless, the animal studies raise serious concern. Therefore, valid arguments can be made to pursue any course of action desired. It is the authors' preference to inform patients about both potential benefits of breastfeeding and risks of AEDs and let the patient help guide the decision. If a woman strongly prefers breastfeeding, then certain measures, discussed next, can be taken to reduce infant exposure. If the woman is risk averse and prefers not to deliver a drug

Table 10.1 Antiepileptic Drugs in Breastfeeding

Antiepileptic Drug	Precautions
Acetazolamide	Limited data are available.
Carbamazepine	Monitor infant for jaundice, drowsiness, poor suckling, vomiting, and poor weight gain.
Clonazepam	Monitor infant for drowsiness.
Diazepam	Avoid repeated doses, if possible.
	Monitor infant for drowsiness.
Eslicarbazepine acetate	No data are available.
	Consider discontinuation of either breastfeeding or eslicarbazepine acetate.
Ethosuximide	Monitor infant for drowsiness, poor suckling, and poor weight gain.
Ezogabine	No data are available.
	Consider discontinuation of either breastfeeding or ezogabine.
Felbamate	No data are available.
Phenobarbital	Monitor infant for drowsiness, poor suckling, and poor weight gain.
	Consider discontinuation of either breastfeeding or phenobarbital.
Phenytoin	Monitor infant for drowsiness and methemoglobinemia.
Primidone	Monitor infant for drowsiness.
Valproic acid	Monitor infant for jaundice and drowsiness.
Gabapentin	Monitor infant for drowsiness.
Lacosamide	No data are available.
	Consider discontinuation of either breastfeeding or lacosamide.
Lamotrigine	Monitor infant for drowsiness.
Levetiracetam	Monitor for drowsiness.
Oxcarbazepine	Monitor infant for drowsiness and lethargy.
Perampanel	No data are available.
Rufinamide	No data are available.
	Consider discontinuation of either breastfeeding or rufinamide.
Tiagabine	No data are available.
Topiramate	Monitor for drowsiness.
	No data are available.
Vigabatrin	Consider discontinuation of either breastfeeding or vigabatrin.
Zonisamide	Monitor for drowsiness.
	No data are available.

that may impair brain development, this becomes obvious during the course of a counseling session.

Should a woman choose to breastfeed, certain advice can be offered. One does not and should not choose an AED for a prospective mother based on breast milk concentration. Therefore, the woman will likely be taking whatever medication was prescribed during pregnancy, and that drug should be continued. Certain medications have more favorable profiles with regard to breast milk concentrations of AEDs. Medications with a short half-life and high degree of protein binding have lower concentrations in breast milk than do drugs with low or intermediate protein binding and longer half-lives (Spencer et al., 2001; Weiner & Buhimschi, 2004; Tomson, 2005). AED concentration in breast milk is roughly inversely proportional to the extent of protein binding of the drug, although significant interindividual variability may exist. Whether lower levels convey less risk is not known, however. Nonetheless, the medication dose should be kept as low as feasible, and breastfeeding should be avoided at times of peak drug levels to minimize dose to the infant. Administer single daily-dose medications just before the longest sleep interval for the infant, usually after the bedtime feeding. Feed infants immediately before medication dose when multiple daily doses are needed. In addition, one can consider using infant formula for some feedings and breast milk for others, to reduce AED delivery (Table 10.1).

References

Bergman A, Feigenbaum JJ, Yanai J. Neuronal losses in mice following both prenatal and neonatal exposure to phenobarbital. *Acta Anatomica (Basel)*. 1982;114: 185–192.

Hall AC, Brennan A, Goold RG, Cleverley K, Lucas FR, Gordon-Weeks PR, Salinas PC. Valproate regulates GSK-3-mediated axonal remodeling and synapsin I clustering in developing neurons. *Mol Cell Neuroscience*. 2002;20: 257–270.

Meador KJ, Baker GA, Browning N, et al. Breastfeeding in children of women taking antiepileptic drugs: cognitive outcomes at age 6 years. *JAMA Pediatr.* 2014;168(8): 729–736.

Patsalos PN, Wiggins RC. Brain maturation following administration of phenobarbital, phenytoin, and sodium valproate to developing rats or to their dams: effects on synthesis of brain myelin and other subcellular membrane proteins. *Journal of Neurochemistry*. 1982;39: 915–923.

Ruiz G, Flores OG, González-Plaza R, Inestrosa NC. Effect of phenytoin on cytoskeletal protein phosphorylation and neuronal structure in the rat sensory cortex. *Journal of Neuroscience Research*. 1987;18: 466–472.

Spencer JP, Gonzalez LS, Barnhart DJ. Medications in the breast-feeding mother. *American Family Physician*. 2001;64: 119–126.

Tomson T. Gender aspects of pharmacokinetics of new and old AEDs: pregnancy and breast-feeding. *Therapeutic Drug Monitoring*. 2005;27: 718–721.

Weiner CP, Buhimschi C. *Drugs for Pregnant and Lactating Women*. Philadelphia: Churchill Livingstone, 2004.

Lundbeck. http://www.sabril.net/2014

Chapter 11

Antiepileptic Drugs in the Elderly

Epilepsy is a common neurological problem in the elderly. The incidence of seizure disorders rises steadily after age 60, so the need for antiepileptic drugs (AEDs) increases with age. Etiologies are diverse. A study of 151 patients with new-onset seizures after age 60 reported that 32% of the seizures were caused by strokes, and 14% were caused by brain tumors. Most tumors were metastatic (71%), and 25% of patients had no identifiable cause (Luhdorf et al., 1986). Other studies have found trauma, infectious causes, toxic and metabolic causes, and degenerative diseases, among others.

While similar principles of drug selection apply to elderly individuals and to younger patients, certain factors carry greater weight in the elderly. Selection of the appropriate therapy should be guided by the recognition that older patients often have comorbidity including neurological disease, receive multiple medications that can affect and be affected by AEDs, and have age-related changes in physiology (e.g., decreased gastrointestinal absorption and renal function). Moreover, elderly individuals may be more sensitive to the adverse effects of AEDs (Perucca et al., 2006; Perucca, 2007). In this age group, monotherapy with an AED is desirable, and lifelong therapy may be required.

Features of AEDs that are especially desirable for use in the elderly include the following:

1. Lack of significant interactions with other medications
2. Lack of induction or inhibition of hepatic microsomal enzymes
3. Minimal protein binding
4. Once- or twice-daily dosing
5. No need for laboratory monitoring
6. Side-effect profile with minimal effects on cognitive function and bone metabolism
7. Low cost

These considerations have practical import. For example, AEDs with enzyme-inducing or inhibiting properties, such as phenobarbital, phenytoin, carbamazepine, primidone, and valproate, alter concentrations of other medications and may render them either less effective or toxic. They also are associated with osteoporosis, which is a significant cause of morbidity in the elderly. The elderly are particularly susceptible to sedating or cognitive adverse effects, so drugs with prominent sedation, such as phenobarbital, benzodiazepines, primidone, and topiramate, may cause greater problems. Because elderly patients are apt to take multiple medications, significant drug-drug interactions that occur with some drugs, such as phenytoin, carbamazepine, phenobarbital, primidone, and valproate, pose a problem. Prolonged exposure to AEDs and potentially interacting drugs may be associated with adverse outcomes such as stroke, myocardial infarction, and mortality. Integrating neurology and clinical pharmacy consultation, combined with electronic medical records systems that alert clinicians to significant drug-drug interactions, may improve care quality and outcomes in this vulnerable population (Pugh et al., 2010). Creatinine clearance (CrCl) is reduced in the elderly, so drugs that are primarily cleared by the kidney such as levetiracetam may accumulate in higher serum concentrations than expected in young patients. These considerations do not mean that drugs that might be more complicated in elderly individuals should not be used but rather that careful attention must be paid to potential interactions, toxic levels, and side effects and that the use of some drugs must be limited, if possible.

Few randomized studies have been performed in older adults comparing different AEDs (Rowan et al., 2005; Saetre et al., 2007), so experience and judgment must play a key role when choosing a drug. The comparison studies performed thus far have compared only lamotrigine, carbamazepine, and gabapentin. Lamotrigine and gabapentin may be somewhat better tolerated than carbamazepine, and while efficacy is similar, there may be a slight advantage of carbamazepine in efficacy over the other drugs. No studies have compared levetiracetam or lacosamide with these drugs, and it is the authors' opinion that these drugs have ideal pharmacological properties and are well suited, perhaps more so than the others, for use in the elderly. The prescribed dose of levetiracetam should be lower in the elderly than in young individuals due to progressively decreasing renal clearance with age.

The following list summarizes features relevant to prescription of AEDs in older patients. Further information regarding relevant pharmacological factors can be found in some of the references (Perucca et al., 2006; *Drug Facts and Comparisons,* 2007, Drugs' websites). In general, when prescribing AEDs to the elderly, start with a lower dose than is used in younger patients, titrate upward more slowly, target a lower final dose, and monitor carefully for side effects because these may appear earlier than usual. Therapeutic monitoring of drug levels may be important for these patients to aid in drug management.

Acetazolamide

Maximum dose in the elderly is similar to that in young adults (*Drug Facts and Comparisons,* 2007). However, dose reductions should be considered in this age group to compensate for age-related reductions in renal drug clearance. There is potential for renal stone formation and drug interaction.

Benzodiazepines

Because elderly patients are more likely to have decreased hepatic and/or renal function, care should be taken in using these drugs and lower doses are used. Observe for sedating effects, and avoid use if possible.

Carbamazepine

Hepatic clearance is decreased by 25%–40% in elderly patients compared with younger adults so lower doses are used (Perucca et al., 2006; Kirmani et al., 2014). Due to drug interactions, use with caution.

Eslicarbazepine

Although the pharmacokinetics of eslicarbazepine are not affected by age independently, dose selection should take into consideration the greater frequency of renal impairment and medical comorbidities and drug therapies in the elderly patient.

Ethosuximide

This drug is rarely appropriate for elderly patients, because they rarely have true absence seizures. Drug interactions are sometimes important.

Ezogabine

Dosage adjustment is recommended in patients aged 65 years and older. Ezogabine may cause urinary retention. Elderly men with symptomatic benign prostatic hyperplasia (BPH) may be at increased risk for urinary retention.

Gabapentin

This is well tolerated and treats concomitant neuropathy and pain. It is often a good choice if these are present. Average decrease in clearance of gabapentin in elderly patients compared with younger adults is about 30%–50%, so lower doses can be used (Perucca et al., 2006). This drug is often a good choice for the elderly, particularly with appropriate comorbidity.

Lacosamide

No dose adjustment based on age is necessary. In elderly patients, dose titration should be performed with caution. This drug is a good choice.

Lamotrigine

The elderly exhibit a reduced hepatic clearance, higher peak concentrations, and longer elimination half-life compared with young adults. Average decrease in apparent clearance of lamotrigine in elderly patients compared with younger adults is about 35% (Perucca et al., 2006). It is recommended that elderly patients receive lower dosages than would be prescribed for young adults, perhaps 150–200 mg daily. This drug is a good choice.

Levetiracetam

This drug has ideal pharmacological properties and is a good choice for elderly patients who require AED therapy. Average decrease in renal clearance of levetiracetam in elderly patients compared with younger adults is about 20%–40% (Perucca et al., 2006), so doses of 500–750 mg daily may be sufficient. This dose is often an excellent choice for the treatment of seizures in the elderly.

Oxcarbazepine

Average decrease in hepatic clearance of oxcarbazepine in elderly patients compared with younger adults is about 25%–35% (Perucca et al., 2006). Adverse effects and drug interactions are relatively favorable; however, hyponatremia is relatively common in our experience. Use with caution because of the potential for hyponatremia.

Perampanel

In elderly patients, dose titration should be performed with caution. An increased risk of falls occurred in patients being treated with perampanel (with and without concurrent seizures). Elderly patients had an increased risk of falls compared to younger adults.

Phenobarbital

Average decrease in hepatic clearance of phenobarbital in elderly patients compared to younger adults is about 20% (Perucca et al., 2006). Due to sedation, hepatic enzyme induction, and drug interactions, limit use. However, this drug is quite inexpensive and may be a reasonable choice when cost poses difficulties (Kirmani et al., 2014). Lower doses, perhaps 45–90 mg daily, are effective in elderly patients.

Phenytoin

Average decrease in hepatic clearance of phenytoin in elderly patients compared with younger adults is about 25% (Perucca et al., 2006). Due to drug interactions and complicated kinetics, this drug is less than ideal. As a cytochrome P-450 enzyme inducer, it increases clearance of other hepatically metabolized drugs and is therefore suboptimal for that reason as well. This is considered a second-line drug, and better choices are available. Cost and ability to give intravenous doses are its major advantages (Kirmani et al., 2014).

Pregabalin

This drug is a reasonable choice for elderly patients, due to minimal drug interactions and treatment of concomitant neuropathy and pain. Reduction of pregabalin dose is required in elderly patients based on CrCl, so that a total dose of 150–200 mg daily may achieve similar levels as higher doses in younger patients.

Primidone

Decreased hepatic clearance mandates lower doses than in young patients. Due to sedative effects, potential for depression, and drug interactions, it should rarely be used. However, if the patient has essential tremor requiring treatment, this drug may treat both conditions.

Rufinamide

In elderly patients, dose titration should be performed with caution. Pharmacokinetics of rufinamide in the elderly is similar to that in young adults.

Tiagabine

Average decrease in clearance of tiagabine in elderly patients compared with younger adults is about 30% (Perucca et al., 2006). Elderly patients may be at increased risk for falls while on this drug (Kirmani et al., 2014). This drug is infrequently used.

Topiramate

The possibility of age-associated renal functional abnormalities should be considered. Average decrease in apparent clearance of topiramate in elderly patients compared to younger adults is about 20% (Perucca et al., 2006). Due to cognitive side effects and potential for renal stones, use with precaution (Kirmani et al., 2014). Comorbidity of migraine and obesity may make this a good choice for some patients. Lower doses, perhaps as low as 50–75 mg per day, may be used.

Valproate

Average decrease in apparent clearance of valproate in elderly patients compared with younger adults is about 40% (Perucca et al., 2006). In addition, a decrease in valproic acid protein binding occurs consequent to hypoalbuminemia, and the half-life of the drug can be prolonged in geriatric patients. In general, use reduced initial dosage and slower dose titration in this age group. Target doses may be as low as 500 mg daily in some patients. Dose reductions or discontinuation should be considered in patients with decreased food or fluid intake and in patients with excessive somnolence.

Zonisamide

Dosage needs to be reduced in elderly patients because of age-related diminished renal clearance. Adverse effects are sometimes important, and the potential for renal stones should be remembered.

Recommended Antiepileptic Drugs in Elderly Persons With Epilepsy

1. **Focal epilepsies:** Lacosamide, lamotrigine, levetiracetam, gabapentin. If cost is a factor, carbamazepine is preferred.
2. **Generalized epilepsies:** These probably do not occur de novo in the elderly but when present consider using lamotrigine or levetiracetam.

References

Drug Facts and Comparisons. St. Louis: Wolters Kluwer Health/Facts & Comparisons, 2007.

Kirmani BF, Robinson DM, Kikam A, Fonkem E, Cruz D. Selection of antiepileptic drugs in older people. *Curr Treat Options Neurol* 2014;16(6): 295.

Luhdorf K, Jensen LK, Plesner AM. Etiology of seizures in the elderly. *Epilepsia*. 1986;27: 458–463.

Perucca E. Age-related changes in pharmacokinetics: predictability and assessment methods. *International Review of Neurobiology*. 2007;81: 183–199.

Perucca E, Berlowitz D, Birnbaum, et al. Pharmacological and clinical aspects of anti-epileptic drug use in the elderly. *Epilepsy Research*. 2006;68S: S49–S63.

Pugh MJ, Vancott AC, Steinman MA, Mortensen EM, Amuan ME, Wang CP, Knoefel JE, Berlowitz DR. Choice of initial antiepileptic drug for older veterans: possible pharmacokinetic drug interactions with existing medications. *J Am Geriatr Soc.* 2010; 58(3): 465–471.

Rowan AJ, Ramsay RE, Collins JF, et al. New onset geriatric epilepsy: a randomized study of gabapentin, lamotrigine, and carbamazepine. *Neurology.* 2005;64: 1868–1873.

Saetre E, Perucca E, Isojärvi J, Gjerstad L, LAM 40089 Study Group. An international multicenter randomized double-blind controlled trial of lamotrigine and sustained-release carbamazepine in the treatment of newly diagnosed epilepsy in the elderly. *Epilepsia.* 2007;48: 1292–1302.

Sunovion. http://www.aptiom.com/2014

Eisai. http://www.banzel.com/2014

GSK. http://www.potiga.com/2014

UCB. http://www.vimpat.com/2014

Eisai. http://www.fycompa.com/2014

Lundbeck. http://www.sabril.net/2014

Chapter 12

Antiepileptic Drugs in Patients With Renal Disease

The use of antiepileptic drugs (AEDs) in the presence of renal insufficiency is associated with an increased risk of adverse effects. Knowledge of the mechanisms of elimination of these drugs is crucial when selecting an AED in epilepsy patients with renal impairment (Kuo et al., 2002; Lacerda et al., 2006; *Drug Facts and Comparisons*, 2007; RxList, n.d.). Drugs that are cleared by the kidneys have different pharmacokinetic properties in the presence of renal failure, and intermittent dialysis can cause significant swings in serum levels, depending on serum levels.

Moreover, renal failure is often accompanied by other medical problems, which can influence drug levels (Kuo et al., 2002). Renal failure is associated with gastroparesis, which slows absorption and bowel edema, which may reduce absorption. There is often a decrease in gut cytochrome P-450 metabolism and P-glycoprotein active transport, which can affect how much of the drug enters the portal circulation. It is also associated with hypoalbuminemia, which may influence free plasma concentrations of AEDs that are highly protein bound. Acidosis may affect albumen-binding affinity as well.

Reduced renal function and hypoalbuminemia lead to accumulation of renally excreted AEDs, such as eslicarbazepine acetate, gabapentin, pregabalin, vigabatrin, and levetiracetam. If there is coexisting impairment of liver function, drugs metabolized by the liver may have altered kinetics as well. AEDs that have low protein binding are largely removed through hemodialysis. Lastly, seizures may be caused by uremia and its associated conditions, such as intracranial hemorrhage, glucose and electrolyte imbalances, dialysis encephalopathy, primary cerebral lymphoma, opportunistic infections, and immunosuppressant toxicity in renal transplant recipients (Kuo et al., 2002).

In patients who require dialysis or in whom dialysis is anticipated, it may be wisest to use drugs that are cleared by hepatic mechanisms rather than eliminated by the kidneys. In addition, AEDs with relatively high levels of protein binding are easier to manage, although they might be less desirable for other properties; a balance must then be struck. Carbamazepine, lamotrigine, benzodiazepines (e.g., clobazam, clonazepam), and rufinamide are preferred when renal failure is present, particularly when dialysis is needed. Therapeutic monitoring of drug levels is important for these patients, and ascertainment of free levels is preferred.

Acetazolamide

Dosage adjustment in patients with renal impairment depends on renal function and creatinine clearance of the patient (Box 12.1).

Intermittent Hemodialysis

Acetazolamide is contraindicated in patients with severe renal disease. It may potentiate acidosis and may cause central nervous system adverse effects in dialysis patients.

Peritoneal Dialysis

Acetazolamide should be avoided in patients on continuous ambulatory peritoneal dialysis to prevent drug-induced hyperkalemia or metabolic acidosis.

Box 12.1 Acetazolamide Dosage Adjustment Based on Renal Function	
Creatinine Clearance (mL/min)	**Dose Regimen**
50 to 80	3 or 4 times/day
10 to 50	1 or 2 times/day
<10	Contraindicated

Benzodiazepines

No quantitative recommendations are available for patients with renal impairment. Due to the lack of renal excretion of unchanged drug, clobazam doses do not need to be adjusted in renal dysfunction. As, active drug is not excreted by the kidneys, clonazepam doses will not need to be reduced in patients with renal dysfunction. The minimal renal excretion of lorazepam, midazolam and diazepam or any of the active metabolites suggests that dosage adjustment is not needed in patients with renal disease (Anderson & Hakimian, 2014).

Carbamazepine

No quantitative recommendations are available for patients with renal impairment. As there is minimal excretion of carbamazepine by the kidneys, carbamazepine doses should not need to be reduced in renal dysfunction (Anderson & Hakimian, 2014).

Eslicarbazepine Acetate

Clearance of eslicarbazepine is decreased in patients with impaired renal function and is correlated with creatinine clearance. Dosage should be modified depending on clinical response and degree of renal impairment. A dose reduction is recommended in patients with renal impairment (creatinine clearance < 60 mL/min). Start treatment at 200 mg once daily. After two weeks, increase dosage to 400 mg once daily, which is the recommended maintenance dosage. Eslicarbazepine is not recommended in patients with creatinine clearance < 30 mL/min. Eslicarbazepine is dialyzable, however, no dosage adjustments have been recommended (Anderson & Hakimian, 2014).

Ethosuximide

No dosage adjustment is needed in patients with renal dysfunction since only a small percentage of ethosuximide is renally eliminated unchanged (Anderson & Hakimian, 2014).

Hemodialysis
Ethosuximide is dialyzable, however, no dosage adjustments have been recommended.

Ezogabine

Dosage adjustment is recommended for patients with creatinine clearance <50 mL/min or patients with end-stage renal disease receiving dialysis treatments. Dosage should be modified depending on clinical response and degree of renal impairment. In patients with renal impairment (CrCL <50 mL/ min or end-stage renal disease on dialysis) the initial dose is 50 mg 3 times daily (150 mg per day) and the maximum dose is 200 mg 3 times daily (600 mg per day). The effect of hemodialysis on ezogabine clearance has not been established.

Felbamate

Felbamate should be used with caution in patients with renal impairment. The starting and maintenance doses should be reduced by one-half in patients with renal impairment.

Gabapentin

Dosage adjustment in patients with renal impairment depends on renal function and CrCl of the patient. The following recommendations (Box 12.2) have been made for adults and adolescents >12 years old.

Intermittent Hemodialysis
Patients on hemodialysis should receive maintenance doses based on CrCl as indicated for patients with renal impairment. A supplemental dose equal to the daily dose plus 50 mg is recommended after a 4-h hemodialysis session (Anderson & Hakimian, 2014).

Box 12.2 Gabapentin Dosage Adjustment Based on Renal Function

Creatinine Clearance (CrCl) (mL/min)	Gabapentin Dosage (mg/day)	Dose Regimen
≥60	900 to 3600	3 times per day
30 to 59	400 to 1400	2 times per day
15 to 29	200 to 700	Once a day
15	100 to 300	Once a day
<15	Reduce daily dose in proportion to CrCl*	Once a day

* For example, patients with a CrCl of 7.5 mL/min should receive one-half the dose that patients with CrCl of 15 mL/min receive.

Lacosamide

No dose adjustment is necessary in patients with mild to moderate renal impairment. A maximum dose of 300 mg per day is recommended for patients with severe renal impairment [CrCl less than or equal to 30 mL/min] and in patients with end-stage renal disease. In all renally impaired patients, the dose titration should be performed with caution. Patients with renal impairment who are taking strong inhibitors of CYP3A4 and CYP2C9 (eg, valproate) may have a significant increase in exposure to lacosamide. Dose reduction may be necessary in these patients.

Intermittent Hemodialysis

Lacosamide is effectively removed from plasma by hemodialysis. Following a 4-hour hemodialysis treatment, dosage supplementation of up to 50% should be considered.

Lamotrigine

In patients with renal impairment, dosage should be modified depending on clinical response and degree of renal impairment. No quantitative recommendations are available.

Intermittent Hemodialysis

Hemodialysis decreases the elimination half-life of lamotrigine. Approximately 20% of lamotrigine present in the body is removed after a standard 4-hour dialysis session (Fillastre et al., 1993). An additional dose of lamotrigine is not needed to maintain therapeutic concentrations (Anderson & Hakimian, 2014). However, adjust dosage schedules to give a normally administered dosage after the hemodialysis session. No quantitative recommendations are available for adjustments.

Levetiracetam

The following dosage adjustments (Box 12.3) pertain to adults with renal impairment using estimated CrCl. Children with renal impairment also need modified dosages but no quantitative recommendations are available.

Intermittent Hemodialysis

Standard hemodialysis results in a roughly 50% clearance of levetiracetam in 4 hours. A supplemental dose (50% of a single usual dose) compensating for this loss is recommended following dialysis.

Box 12.3 Levetiracetam Dosage Adjustment Based on Renal Function		
Creatinine Clearance (mL/min)	Levetiracetam Dosage (mg/day)	Dose Regimen
>80	No need for adjustment	—
50 to 80	1000 to 2000	2 times per day
30 to 49	500 to 1500	2 times per day
<30	500 to 1000	2 times per day

Oxcarbazepine

If CrCl >30 mL/min, no dosage adjustments have been recommended. However, renal clearance of MHD, the active metabolite, declines linearly with a decrease in creatinine clearance. If CrCl <30 mL/min, renal clearance of MHD is decreased. Therefore, initiate therapy with 50% of the usual starting dose and slowly titrate upward as necessary.

Perampanel

No dosage adjustment is necessary for patients with mild renal impairment. Perampanel can be used in patients with moderate renal impairment with close monitoring. A slower titration may be considered based on clinical response and tolerability. Use in patients with severe renal impairment or patients undergoing hemodialysis is not recommended.

Phenobarbital

If CrCl >10 mL/min, no dosage adjustment is needed. If CrCl <10 mL/min, significantly decrease dosage by increasing the interval between the doses to

12 hours or longer. Adjust dosage based on clinical response and serum concentrations. The chronic use of phenobarbital should generally be avoided in patients with renal failure.

Intermittent Hemodialysis

Phenobarbital is efficiently removed through hemodialysis. Adjust dosage schedules to give a normally administered dosage after the hemodialysis session. It is better to administer the supplementary dose after hemodialysis.

Peritoneal Dialysis

Peritoneal dialysis (as CAPD) removes phenobarbital by almost 35%–50% (not as efficient as hemodialysis) (Porto et al., 1997). No quantitative recommendations for dose adjustment are available. Some references have suggested that 50% of a normal dose be given after a CAPD session.

Phenytoin

If CrCl >10 mL/min, no dosage adjustment is needed. If CrCl <10 mL/min, dosage adjustment and serum concentration monitoring are necessary. Decreased protein binding occurs in uremia, and the unbound (free) fraction of phenytoin may be increased. Dosing adjustments may be required based on serum free phenytoin level monitoring and clinical response.

Dialysis (Hemodialysis or Peritoneal Dialysis)

Phenytoin is not significantly removed during a standard hemodialysis session or continuous hemodialysis or peritoneal dialysis. However, supplemental dosing after dialysis is controversial.

Pregabalin

Dose adjustments are required in patients with renal impairment with CrCl <60 mL/min (Box 12.4). Reduction of pregabalin dose may be required in elderly patients based on CrCl.

Box 12.4 Pregabalin Dosage Adjustment Based on Renal Function		
Creatinine Clearance (mL/min)	**Pregabalin Dosage (mg/day)**	**Dose Regimen**
>60	No need for adjustment	—
30 to 60	75 to 300	2 or 3 divided doses
15 to 30	25 to 150	1 or 2 times per day
<15	25 to 75	Once per day

Intermittent Hemodialysis

Pregabalin is effectively removed through hemodialysis because it has little plasma protein binding. Each 4-hour hemodialysis session removes 50%–60% of the amount of drug present in the circulation in patients on three-times-per-week hemodialysis. For patients undergoing hemodialysis, pregabalin daily dose should be adjusted based on renal function. In addition to the daily dose adjustment, a supplemental (single additional) dose should be given immediately following every 4-hour hemodialysis treatment as follows:

- **Patients on the 25 mg/day regimen:** Take one supplemental dose of 25 mg or 50 mg.
- **Patients on the 25–50 mg/day regimen:** Take one supplemental dose of 50 mg or 75 mg.
- **Patients on the 50–70 mg/day regimen:** Take one supplemental dose of 75 mg or 100 mg.
- **Patients on the 75 mg/day regimen:** Take one supplemental dose of 100 mg or 150 mg.

Primidone

Dose adjustments are required in patients with renal impairment with CrCl <50 mL/min (Box 12.5). Monitor clinical response and serum concentrations.

Intermittent Hemodialysis

Primidone is partially removed through hemodialysis. Some references recommend supplementing with one-third of a routine dose after a hemodialysis session. We generally avoid prescribing this drug irrespective of diagnosis.

Box 12.5 Primidone Dosage Adjustment Based on Renal Function	
Creatinine Clearance (mL/min)	**Dose Regimen**
>50	No dosage adjustment is needed
10 to 50	Every 8 to 12 hours
<10	Every 12 to 24 hours

Rufinamide

Renally impaired patients (CrCl < 30 mL/min) do not require any special dosage change. Rufinamide pharmacokinetics in patients with severe renal impairment (CrCl <30 mL/min) was similar to that of healthy subjects.

Intermittent Hemodialysis

Patients undergoing dialysis 3 hours post-rufinamide dosing showed a reduction in AUC and Cmax by 29% and 16%, respectively. Adjusting rufinamide dose for the loss of drug upon dialysis should be considered. No quantitative recommendations are available for adjustments.

Tiagabine

No initial dosage adjustment is required in patients with renal impairment. Adjust dosage according to patient's response and tolerance.

Topiramate

In adults, if CrCl <70 mL/min, reduce the topiramate dose to one-half of the usual dose. In children, adjustment may be required but should be individualized because clearance rates are higher in children than in adults. Patients with renal impairment may require a longer time than patients with normal renal function to reach steady state with each topiramate dosage adjustment.

Intermittent Hemodialysis

During the hemodialysis session, adult patients clear topiramate at a rate that is 4–6 times greater than that of an adult person with normal renal function. A supplemental dose of topiramate may be required during or after hemodialysis.

Valproate

In patients with severe renal impairment or renal failure, uremia can cause an increase in the free fraction of the drug, resulting in possible toxicity. Also, unbound valproic acid in the blood may be cleared more rapidly than bound drug. Close monitoring of valproic acid serum concentrations may be warranted to ensure adequate dosage, ensure efficacy, and limit toxicity. A supplemental dose of valproate may be required after hemodialysis in some patients.

Vigabatrin

There are no published studies on the effect of renal dysfunction on vigabatrin pharmacokinetics. It is recommended that the dose of vigabatrin be reduced by 25%, 50%, or 75% for patients with mild (CrCl 50–80 mL/min), moderate (CrCl 30–50 mL/min), or severe (CrCl 10–30 mL/min) renal dysfunction.

Zonisamide

Because zonisamide is excreted by the kidneys, patients with renal impairment or renal disease should be treated with caution. Slower titration and more frequent monitoring may be required. No quantitative recommendations are available.

Intermittent Hemodialysis

Zonisamide is partially removed through hemodialysis (about 50%). Adjust dosage schedules to give a normally administered dosage after the hemodialysis session.

Recommended Antiepileptic Drugs in Epilepsy Patients With Renal Failure

1. **Generalized epilepsies:** Clobazam, ethosuximide, lamotrigine, rufinamide (in patients with Lennox-Gastaut syndrome)
2. **Focal epilepsies:** Carbamazepine, clobazam, lamotrigine, phenytoin

Note: Seizures are a serious complication of hemodialysis in people with epilepsy. They may occur within the first 24 hours of beginning dialysis and are usually tonic-clonic. Preexisting hypertension and the use of dialyzable anticonvulsant drugs are associated with dialysis-related seizures. They may be due to the removal of these drugs at a time when metabolic stress induces seizures.

In one pediatric study, phenobarbital was given at a dosage of 5 mg/kg/day orally twice daily to prevent dialysis-associated seizures. Also, diazepam (0.5 mg/kg orally) was administered 30 minutes before each dialysis session in some patients. Patients receiving diazepam prophylaxis had significantly fewer seizures than those with no treatment or patients receiving phenobarbital alone. Therefore, administration of oral diazepam, a nondialyzable anticonvulsant drug, 30 minutes before each dialysis, may help prevent seizure recurrence (Sonmez et al., 2000).

Urinary Adverse Effects of Antiepileptic Drugs (Lacerda et al., 2006; *Drug Facts and Comparisons*, 2007; RxList, n.d.)

Acetazolamide
Carbonic anhydrase inhibitors are sulfonamide derivatives that have caused crystalluria and sulfonamide-like nephrotoxicity characterized by renal tubular obstruction, hematuria, dysuria, and oliguria. An increase in calcium excretion can cause nephrolithiasis. Patients with preexisting hypercalcemia develop renal calculi most frequently.

Benzodiazepines
No significant urinary adverse effects have been reported.

Carbamazepine
Urinary side effects include increased urinary frequency, acute urinary retention, oliguria with elevated blood pressure, azotemia, and renal failure. Albuminuria, glycosuria, and microscopic deposits in the urine have also been observed. Antidiuretic effects and hyponatremia have been reported.

Carbamazepine may rarely cause interstitial nephritis or other renal diseases. Occasional monitoring of renal parameters or urinalysis has been recommended.

Eslicarbazepine acetate

No significant urinary adverse effects have been reported.

Ethosuximide

No significant urinary adverse effects have been reported.

Ezogabine

Because of the increased risk of urinary retention on ezogabine (in about 2% of the patients), urologic symptoms should be carefully monitored. Urinary retention was generally reported within the first 6 months of treatment, but was also observed later. Closer monitoring is recommended for patients who have other risk factors for urinary retention (e.g., benign prostatic hyperplasia), patients who are unable to communicate clinical symptoms (e.g., cognitively impaired patients), or patients who use concomitant medications that may affect voiding (e.g., anticholinergics). In these patients, a comprehensive evaluation of urologic symptoms prior to and during treatment with ezogabine may be appropriate. Hydronephrosis is a rare adverse effect in patients taking ezogabine. Dysuria and hematuria have been reported as adverse effects of ezogabine.

Felbamate

Crystalluria and urolithiasis have been reported with felbamate. Urinary tract infection and lowered blood urea nitrogen levels have been reported as a result of felbamate therapy.

Gabapentin

No significant urinary adverse effects have been reported.

Lacosamide

No significant urinary adverse effects have been reported.

Lamotrigine

No significant urinary adverse effects have been reported.

Levetiracetam

No significant urinary adverse effects have been reported.

Oxcarbazepine

Dysuria, hematuria, increased urinary frequency, urinary tract pain, polyuria, and renal calculus have been reported as adverse effects of oxcarbazepine.

Perampanel

No significant urinary adverse effects have been reported.

Phenobarbital

No significant urinary adverse effects have been reported. Reports of interstitial nephritis are rare.

Phenytoin

Phenytoin rarely causes renal complications. Glomerulonephritis, interstitial nephritis, proteinuria, and nephrotic syndrome have been reported.

Pregabalin

There are reports of increased urinary frequency and urinary incontinence with pregabalin. However, causality between pregabalin and these adverse events has not been definitively established.

Rufinamide

Urinary incontinence, dysuria, hematuria, nephrolithiasis, polyuria, enuresis, nocturia, and incontinence have infrequently been reported as adverse effects of rufinamide.

Tiagabine

No significant urinary adverse effects have been reported.

Topiramate

Nephrolithiasis, hematuria, increased urinary frequency, dysuria, and urinary incontinence have been reported as adverse effects of topiramate.

Valproate

No significant urinary adverse effects have been reported.

Vigabatrin

No significant urinary adverse effects have been reported.

Zonisamide

Increases in serum creatinine and blood urea nitrogen have been reported. Nephrolithiasis has been reported in some patients. Other infrequent adverse reactions affecting the urinary system in zonisamide-treated patients include dysuria, hematuria, nocturia, polyuria, urinary frequency, urinary incontinence, urinary retention, and urinary urgency. Rare adverse reactions include albuminuria, bladder pain, and bladder calculus.

Renal Stones

Zonisamide, topiramate, and acetazolamide, which all have carbonic anhydrase-inhibiting properties, are associated with a modest increase in the incidence of renal stones due to reduced urinary citrate excretion and increased urinary pH. Zonisamide is associated with a 4% incidence of renal stones. Approximately 1.5% of patients treated with topiramate developed kidney stones compared with the annual 0.5% incidence of renal stones in the general population. Men are at higher risk for kidney stones, and the association has also been reported for children treated with topiramate. The analyzed stones are mainly composed of calcium phosphate (Kuo et al., 2002). The ketogenic diet may also be associated with renal stones (Kossoff et al., 2002).

In general, increasing fluid intake and urine output can help reduce the risk of stone formation in patients taking zonisamide, topiramate, or acetazolamide or those on the ketogenic diet, particularly in patients with predisposing factors (Kossoff et al., 2002). If there is marked benefit with therapy with one of these drugs, and drugs that do not cause nephrolithiasis have not proved effective, the development of renal calculi is not an absolute indication to discontinue the treatment (Richards et al., 2005).

References

Anderson GD, Hakimian S. Pharmacokinetic of antiepileptic drugs in patients with hepatic or renal impairment. *Clin Pharmacokinet.* 2014;53(1): 29–49.

Drug Facts and Comparisons. St. Louis: Wolters Kluwer Health/Facts & Comparisons, 2007.

Fillastre JP, Taburet AM, Fialaire A, et al. Pharmacokinetics of lamotrigine in patients with renal impairment: influence of haemodialysis. *Drugs Under Experimental and Clinical Research.* 1993;19: 25–32.

Kossoff EH, Pyzik PL, Furth SL, et al. Kidney stones, carbonic anhydrase inhibitors, and the ketogenic diet. *Epilepsia.* 2002;43: 1168–1171.

Kuo RL, Moran ME, Kim DH, et al. Topiramate-Induced nephrolithiasis. *Journal of Endocrinology.* 2002;16: 229–231.

Lacerda G, Krummel T, Sabourdy C, et al. Optimizing therapy of seizures in patients with renal or hepatic dysfunction. *Neurology.* 2006;67: S28–S33.

Porto I, John EG, Heilliczer J. Removal of phenobarbital during continuous cycling peritoneal dialysis in a child. *Pharmacotherap.* 1997;17: 832–835.

Richards KC, Smith MC, Verma A. Continued use of zonisamide following development of renal calculi. *Neurology.* 2005;64: 763–764.

RxList: *The Internet drug list.* Retrieved from RxList Inc. http://www.rxlist.com/2014.

Sonmez F, Mir S, Tutuncuoglu S. Potential prophylactic use of benzodiazepines for hemodialysis-associated seizures. *Pediatric Nephrology.* 2000;14: 367–369.

Sunovion. http://www.aptiom.com/2014

Eisai. http://www.banzel.com/2014

GSK. http://www.potiga.com/2014

UCB. http://www.vimpat.com/2014

Eisai. http://www.fycompa.com/2014

Lundbeck. http://www.sabril.net/2014

Chapter 13

Antiepileptic Drugs in Patients With Liver Disease

The use of antiepileptic drugs (AEDs) in the presence of liver diseases and hepatic dysfunction is associated with an increased risk of adverse effects. Knowledge of the mechanisms of metabolism and elimination of these drugs is crucial when selecting an AED in epilepsy patients with liver disease. Loss of hepatocytes and disruption of liver blood flow may alter the metabolism of some AEDs. Hypoalbuminemia and impaired metabolism by cytochrome P-450 and glucuronyl transferase enzymes may increase free AED levels (Lacerda et al., 2006). The type of hepatic disease may also preferentially affect some enzyme systems; for example, CYP3A4 is affected more in hepatocellular dysfunction, and CYP2E1 is affected more in cholestasis. Unlike renal failure, which can be quantified, liver disease is not easily quantifiable, so adjustments in dosing are more difficult. Fortunately, even moderate liver dysfunction does not significantly impact AED clearance, other than problems caused by associated hypoalbuminemia, so dose adjustments are usually needed until hepatic dysfunction is severe. In addition, some AEDs have important hepatic adverse effects (Lacerda et al., 2006; *Drug Facts and Comparisons*, 2007). Last, hepatic failure may cause renal impairment, so kidney function needs to be monitored and AED dosing adjusted accordingly. Therapeutic monitoring of drug levels is important for these patients, and ascertainment of free levels is preferred.

In general, drugs cleared by the kidneys are preferred for ease of management and reduced incidence of adverse effects, such as levetiracetam, gabapentin, and pregabalin, while valproate, phenytoin, phenobarbital, and carbamazepine are less desirable.

Acetazolamide

Avoid acetazolamide use in patients with hepatic impairment. Patients with hepatic disease (e.g., cirrhosis) are at increased risk for hepatic encephalopathy and electrolyte imbalances (e.g., hypokalemia) (Lacerda et al., 2006; *Drug Facts and Comparisons*, 2007).

Benzodiazepines

These drugs are to be avoided if possible. Dosage should be modified depending on clinical response and degree of hepatic impairment, but no quantitative recommendations are available for benzodiazepines. Hepatic dysfunction is among the adverse effects reported.

Clonazepam undergoes hepatic metabolism, and liver disease may impair clonazepam elimination. The drug should not be used in patients with significant liver dysfunction.

Lorazepam undergoes glucuronidation in the liver to inactive metabolites. However, studies in patients with cirrhosis or other significant liver diseases did not note a need for dose reduction (Lacerda et al., 2006; *Drug Facts and Comparisons*, 2007). Therefore, lorazepam may be the benzodiazepine of choice (if there is no other alternative) for patients with liver disease since its half-life is minimally increased in the presence of hepatic dysfunction.

Carbamazepine

Carbamazepine is not recommended in patients with decompensated liver disease. Dose reductions may be necessary in patients with stable hepatic disease.

Various hepatic adverse effects may occur during carbamazepine treatment, ranging from asymptomatic elevated liver enzymes to more serious derangements. Hepatitis and cholestasis have rarely been reported with carbamazepine therapy. Consider discontinuation of the drug if newly occurring or worsening clinical or laboratory evidences of liver dysfunction or hepatic damage occur during carbamazepine treatment (Lacerda et al., 2006; *Drug Facts and Comparisons*, 2007).

Eslicarbazepine Acetate

Dose adjustments are not required in patients with mild to moderate hepatic impairment. Use of eslicarbazepine acetate in patients with severe hepatic impairment has not been studied and is not recommended.

Hepatic effects, ranging from mild to moderate elevations in transaminases to rare cases with concomitant elevations of total bilirubin have been reported with eslicarbazepine acetate use. The combination of transaminase elevations and elevated bilirubin without evidence of obstruction is generally recognized as an important predictor of severe liver injury. Eslicarbazepine acetate should be discontinued in patients with jaundice or other evidence of significant liver injury (http://www.aptiom.com).

Ethosuximide

Specific guidelines for dosage adjustments of ethosuximide in hepatic impairment are not available. Dosage adjustment may be needed in moderate and severe cirrhosis and ethosuximide plasma concentrations should be monitored (Anderson & Hakimian, 2014).

Elevated hepatic enzymes have been reported with ethosuximide treatment. Serious hepatic dysfunction may be an indication of drug hypersensitivity reaction and may require drug discontinuation (Knowles et al., 1999; Lacerda et al., 2006; *Drug Facts and Comparisons*, 2007).

Ezogabine

No dosage adjustment is required for patients with mild hepatic impairment. In patients with moderate or severe hepatic impairment, the initial and maintenance dosage of ezogabine should be reduced. In patients with hepatic impairment and Child-Pugh 7-9, the initial dose is 50 mg 3 times daily (150 mg/day) and the maximum dose is 250 mg 3 times daily (750 mg/day). In patients with hepatic impairment and Child-Pugh >9, the initial dose is 50 mg 3 times daily (150 mg/day) and the maximum dose is 200 mg 3 times daily (600 mg/day). Elevated hepatic enzymes have been reported with ezogabine treatment (http://www.potiga.com).

Felbamate

Felbamate may cause idiosyncratic hepatotoxicity and massive hepatic necrosis (O'Neil et al., 1996). Felbamate may be contraindicated in patients with a history of hepatic impairment, although there are little data to support this recommendation. *It should be used only in the treatment of severe epilepsy refractory to other AEDs because of the risk of acute liver failure.* Patients or their caregivers should be advised of the symptoms of liver disease. Liver function tests are recommended before beginning treatment and regularly during treatment. Felbamate should be stopped if there is any evidence of liver abnormalities (Lacerda et al., 2006; *Drug Facts and Comparisons*, 2007).

Gabapentin

No dosage adjustment is necessary in patients with hepatic impairment, since gabapentin is not metabolized by the liver. Hepatic adverse effects have rarely been reported (Lacerda et al., 2006; *Drug Facts and Comparisons*, 2007).

Lacosamide

The dose titration should be performed with caution in patients with hepatic impairment. A maximum dose of 300 mg/day is recommended for patients with mild or moderate hepatic impairment. Lacosamide use is not recommended in patients with severe hepatic impairment. Patients with hepatic impairment who are taking strong inhibitors of CYP3A4 and CYP2C9 (e.g., valproate) may have a significant increase in exposure to lacosamide. Dose reduction may be necessary in these patients. Elevated hepatic enzymes have been reported with lacosamide treatment (http://www.vimpat.com).

Lamotrigine

Initial escalation and maintenance doses should be reduced by approximately 50% in patients with moderate hepatic impairment (Child-Pugh Grade B) and 75% in patients with severe (Child-Pugh Grade C) hepatic impairment. Doses of lamotrigine should be reduced by one- third in patients with Gilbert's syndrome. Adjust doses as needed according to clinical response. Abnormal liver function tests have been reported with lamotrigine treatment (Lacerda et al., 2006; *Drug Facts and Comparisons*, 2007; Anderson & Hakimian, 2014).

Levetiracetam

No dosage adjustment is necessary in patients with mild to moderate hepatic impairment. Levetiracetam is not extensively metabolized by the liver. The dose of levetiracetam should be reduced by 50% in patients with severe hepatic dysfunction (Lacerda et al., 2006; *Drug Facts and Comparisons*, 2007; Anderson & Hakimian, 2014).

Oxcarbazepine

No dosage adjustments are recommended for mild to moderate hepatic impairment. The effects of severe hepatic impairment have not been evaluated. Hepatic adverse effects have rarely been reported with oxcarbazepine treatment. Abnormal liver function tests have been reported (Lacerda et al., 2006; *Drug Facts and Comparisons*, 2007).

Perampanel

Because perampanel has higher exposure and longer half-life in patients with mild and moderate hepatic impairment, dosage adjustment is recommended. Starting dose should be 2 mg/day, with weekly increments of 2 mg/day every 2 weeks until target dose is achieved. The maximum recommended daily dose is 6 mg for patients with mild hepatic impairment and 4 mg for patients with moderate hepatic impairment. Dose increases in patients with mild and moderate hepatic impairment, as with all patients, should be based on clinical response and tolerability. Use in patients with severe hepatic impairment is not recommended (http://www.fycompa.com/2014).

Phenobarbital/Primidone

These drugs should be avoided in patients with hepatic disease, due to sedative effects and decreased protein binding. Modify initial dose depending on degree of hepatic impairment. A 50% reduction in dose may be needed in patients with moderate to severe hepatic cirrhosis. Initiate phenobarbital cautiously and adjust the dose based on clinical response and serum concentrations. Hepatic adverse effects have rarely been reported. Because of sedating effects, it may precipitate coma in hepatic encephalopathy and is not recommended (Lacerda et al., 2006; *Drug Facts and Comparisons*, 2007; Anderson & Hakimian, 2014).

Phenytoin

Phenytoin is primarily metabolized in the liver, and patients with hepatic disease may rapidly show signs of phenytoin toxicity. In addition, serum concentrations of free phenytoin may be increased due to hypoalbuminemia that is commonly present in cirrhotic liver diseases. Dosing adjustments may be required based on serum phenytoin level monitoring and clinical response.

Phenytoin is potentially hepatotoxic. It can cause elevated hepatic enzymes or more serious manifestations of hepatitis such as focal hepatic necrosis and hepatomegaly. Cholestasis with jaundice can occur. Hepatotoxicity may also be a component of a severe hypersensitivity reaction (antiepileptic hypersensitivity syndrome) (Knowles et al., 1999). Careful investigation should be considered in case of any evidence suggestive of hepatic injury (Lacerda et al., 2006; *Drug Facts and Comparisons*, 2007).

Pregabalin

This drug is cleared by the kidneys and has low protein binding. No dosage adjustments are required (Lacerda et al., 2006; *Drug Facts and Comparisons*, 2007).

Rufinamide

Use of rufinamide in patients with hepatic impairment has not been studied. Therefore, use in patients with severe hepatic impairment is not recommended. Caution should be exercised in treating patients with mild to moderate hepatic impairment (http://www.banzel.com).

Tiagabine

Because the half-life of tiagabine is prolonged in patients with hepatic disease, dosage reduction and longer dosing intervals may be necessary. However, specific dosing guidelines have not been established (Lacerda et al., 2006; *Drug Facts and Comparisons*, 2007).

Topiramate

While mostly excreted by the kidneys, topiramate is partially metabolized by the liver. In liver failure, topiramate half-life may be lengthened, and dosage reduction may be required. Elevated hepatic enzymes, hepatic failure, and hepatitis have been rarely reported with topiramate treatment (Lacerda et al., 2006; *Drug Facts and Comparisons*, 2007). Topiramate (as well as potentially other drugs with carbonic anhydrase activity such as zonisamide and acetazolamide) may affect the clearance of ammonia via their effects on renal carbonic anhydrase activity, leading to worsening hepatic encephalopathy (Anderson & Hakimian, 2014).

Valproate

Drug clearance may be decreased by 50% in cirrhosis, because it is cleared by the liver. Therefore, dosage reductions may be required in hepatic failure. There is no compelling evidence that patients with liver disease are at greater risk for valproate-induced hepatotoxicity than other individuals.

In rare cases, valproate may cause liver failure, mainly in children. Hepatotoxicity due to valproate is most likely to occur within the first 6 months of treatment. Idiosyncratic hepatotoxicity is rare and not predictable on the basis of laboratory monitoring. Risk factors for hepatotoxicity include

- children, especially those less than 2 years of age
- patients receiving multiple AEDs
- patients with other complicating factors (e.g., metabolic diseases, mental retardation, and organic brain syndromes)
- mitochondrial disease

Because liver dysfunction associated with valproic acid is likely dose related, titrate dose slowly in susceptible patients. Changes in hepatic function may be indicated by loss of seizure control, jaundice, malaise, weakness, lethargy, facial edema, anorexia, or vomiting. The most serious adverse reaction induced by valproic acid is hepatic failure. There are some data that support the hypothesis that L-carnitine treatment improves survival of patients with severe valproate-induced hepatotoxicity (Fenichel and Greene, 1985; Verrotti et al., 2002; Lacerda et al., 2006; *Drug Facts and Comparisons*, 2007).

Vigabatrin

Vigabatrin is not significantly metabolized. With negligible protein binding and minimal to no hepatic metabolism, dose adjustment is not necessary in hepatic diseases. It should be used only in the treatment of severe epilepsy refractory to other AEDs because of the risk of visual field defect.

Vigabatrin decreases alanine transaminase (ALT) and aspartate transaminase (AST) plasma activity in up to 90% of patients. In some patients, these enzymes become undetectable. The suppression of ALT and AST activity may preclude the use of these markers to detect early hepatic injury (http://www.sabril.net/2014).

Zonisamide

Because zonisamide is hepatically metabolized, patients with hepatic disease should be treated with caution. Slower titration and more frequent monitoring may be required. However, no quantitative recommendations are available.

Elevated hepatic enzymes, hepatitis, fulminant hepatic necrosis, cholangitis, and cholecystitis have been rarely reported with zonisamide treatment (Lacerda et al., 2006; *Drug Facts and Comparisons*, 2007).

Recommended Antiepileptic Drugs in Epilepsy Patients With Liver Disease

1. **Generalized epilepsies:** Levetiracetam
2. **Focal epilepsies:** Gabapentin, levetiracetam, oxcarbazepine, pregabalin, vigabatrin (only for patients who are refractory to all other options)

References

Anderson GD, Hakimian S. Pharmacokinetic of antiepileptic drugs in patients with hepatic or renal impairment. *Clin Pharmacokinet* 2014;53(1): 29–49.

Drug Facts and Comparisons. St. Louis: Wolters Kluwer Health/Facts & Comparisons, 2007.

Fenichel GM, Greene HL. Valproate hepatotoxicity: two new cases, a summary of others, and recommendations. *Pediatric Neurology*. 1985;1: 109–113.

Knowles SR, Shapiro LE, Shear NH. Anticonvulsant hypersensitivity syndrome: incidence, prevention and management. *Drug Safety*. 1999;21: 489–501.

Lacerda G, Krummel T, Sabourdy C, Ryvlin P, Hirsch E. Optimizing therapy of seizures in patients with renal or hepatic dysfunction. *Neurology*. 2006;67: S28–S33.

O'Neil MG, Perdun CS, Wilson MB, et al. Felbamate-associated fatal acute hepatic necrosis. *Neurology*. 1996;46: 1457–1459.

Verrotti A, Trota D, Morgese G, Chiarelli F. Valproate-induced hyperammonemic encephalopathy. *Metabolic Brain Diseases*. 2002;17: 367–373.

Sunovion. http://www.aptiom.com/2014

Eisai. http://www.banzel.com/2014

GSK. http://www.potiga.com/2014

UCB. http://www.vimpat.com/2014

Eisai. http://www.fycompa.com/2014

Lundbeck. http://www.sabril.net/2014

Chapter 14

Antiepileptic Drugs and Metabolic Disorders

Metabolic Acidosis

Three antiepileptic drugs (AEDs)—acetazolamide, topiramate, and zonisamide—are typically associated with metabolic acidosis due to their property of inhibiting the enzyme carbonic anhydrase. All are associated with various degrees of renal tubular acidosis (Sheth, 2004).

Topiramate is associated with a mild hyperchloremic, non–anion gap metabolic acidosis manifest by a persistently low bicarbonate level. Bicarbonate decrements are usually mild to moderate, with an average decrease of 4 mEq/L at daily doses of 400 mg in adults and approximately 6 mg/kg/day in pediatric patients. Decreases of more than 10 mEq/L can be found in rare cases. The metabolic acidosis typically occurs soon after initiation of therapy. Conditions or therapies that predispose to acidosis such as renal disease, severe respiratory disorders, status epilepticus, diarrhea, surgery, ketogenic diet, or other drugs may add to the bicarbonate-lowering effects of topiramate.

Baseline and periodic measurements of serum bicarbonate levels during topiramate, zonisamide, and acetazolamide treatment are recommended, especially in children. If metabolic acidosis develops and persists, consideration should be given to reducing the dosage or discontinuing these AEDs, especially topiramate, considering the adverse effects of chronic metabolic acidosis on kidney, bone, heart, and growth (in children). If the decision is made to continue topiramate therapy despite persistent acidosis, alkali treatment should be considered (Sheth, 2004; Groeper and McCann, 2005).

It is reasonable to avoid prescribing these three AEDs (acetazolamide, topiramate, and zonisamide) in patients with preexisting disorders with metabolic acidosis (e.g., inborn errors of metabolism, renal tubular acidosis, etc.).

Hyponatremia

Hyponatremia occurs in patients treated with carbamazepine, oxcarbazepine, or eslicarbazepine acetate. In most patients, the hyponatremia is transient, mild, and asymptomatic. However, in one recent study, it was observed that mild hyponatremia is associated with an increased risk of death in an ambulatory setting (Gankam-Kengne et al., 2013).

Hyponatremia occurs more frequently with oxcarbazepine than with carbamazepine. This adverse effect typically occurs during the first 3 months of treatment; rare cases of symptomatic hyponatremia beginning more than 1 year after treatment initiation have been observed. The mechanism by which carbamazepine and oxcarbazepine cause hyponatremia is not completely understood. Patients typically present with findings similar to the syndrome of inappropriate secretion of antidiuretic hormone (SIADH) (Asconapé, 2002). However, a mechanism other than SIADH may be partially responsible, because some cases of hyponatremia without abnormal ADH levels have been observed (Sachdeo et al., 2002). The risk of developing significant hyponatremia with the use of oxcarbazepine is age related, more common in the elderly (Dong et al., 2005). In a study of 97 oxcarbazepine-treated and 451 carbamazepine-treated patients (Dong et al., 2005), the prevalence of hyponatremia, defined as serum sodium less than 134 mEq/L, was 29.9% among oxcarbazepine-treated patients and 13.5% among carbamazepine-treated patients. Severe hyponatremia, defined by the authors as serum sodium less than 128 mEq/L, was found in 12.4% of oxcarbazepine-treated patients and 2.8% of carbamazepine-treated patients.

Periodic monitoring of sodium levels is recommended during the first 3 months of therapy with oxcarbazepine in elderly patients, patients with renal failure, and patients on other medications associated with hyponatremia. Patients with stable sodium levels above 130 mEq/L during the first 3 months are at minimal risk for late development of hyponatremia, and no further monitoring is usually necessary. In patients with sodium levels between 125 and 130 mEq/L, repeat measurements are recommended to confirm that hyponatremia is not worsening. When the serum sodium level falls below 125 mEq/L or hyponatremic symptoms appear, intervention is necessary, consisting either of water restriction or change in medication (Asconapé, 2002).

Clinically significant hyponatremia (sodium <125 mEq/L) can develop in patients taking eslicarbazepine acetate. This effect is dose related and generally appears within the first 8 weeks of treatment (as early as after 3 days). Serious, life-threatening complications were reported with eslicarbazepine-associated hyponatremia (as low as 112 mEq/L) including seizures and severe nausea/vomiting leading to dehydration. Concurrent hypochloremia was also present in patients with hyponatremia. Depending on the severity of hyponatremia, the dose of eslicarbazepine may need to be reduced or discontinued. Measurement of serum sodium and chloride levels should be considered during maintenance treatment with eslicarbazepine, particularly if the patient is receiving other medications known to decrease serum sodium levels and should be performed if symptoms of hyponatremia develop (e.g., nausea/vomiting, malaise, headache, lethargy, confusion, irritability, muscle weakness/spasms, obtundation, or increase in seizure frequency or severity).

Oligohidrosis

Cases of oligohidrosis, hyperthermia, and heat stroke have been reported with topiramate and zonisamide. All patients with dehydration, hypovolemia, or other predisposing factors to heat intolerance should have their condition corrected before using topiramate or zonisamide. All patients, especially children, should be instructed to limit exposure to high temperatures. The concurrent use of drugs that predispose patients to heat intolerance, such as anticholinergic medications and carbonic anhydrase inhibitors, should be avoided when topiramate and zonisamide are taken. To help prevent oligohidrosis and hyperthermia in patients treated with either drug, proper hydration is suggested before and during strenuous activity or exposure to warm temperatures (*Drug Facts and Comparisons*, 2007).

Hyperammonemia

Hyperammonemia can occur in as many as half of patients receiving valproic acid, regardless of liver function status. In most patients, elevated ammonia levels are minimal and benign, but in some patients, lethargy and/or coma have been reported. Early recognition of subtle cognitive and behavioral changes in patients taking valproate and early therapeutic interventions may prevent the development of more severe problems. There are some preliminary data that support the hypothesis that L-carnitine treatment significantly enhances the survival of these patients (Verrotti et al., 2002). If symptomatic hyperammonemia occurs, L-carnitine at a dosage of 330–990 mg three times daily can be given, usually with prompt resolution of symptoms.

Patients with *urea cycle disorders (UCD)* should not receive valproate. These individuals have a genetic enzyme defect leading to an impaired ability to produce urea. Hyperammonemic encephalopathy has been reported following initiation of valproate therapy in patients with UCD (Thakur et al., 2006). Similarly, patients with a known mitochondrial disorder should not receive valproate, because it may cause liver failure.

Hyperammonemia and encephalopathy are reported with concomitant valproic acid and topiramate use in patients who have tolerated either drug alone. Clinical symptoms include acute alteration in level of consciousness and/or cognitive function with lethargy or vomiting. In most patients, symptoms and signs abated with discontinuation of either drug (*Drug Facts and Comparisons*, 2007).

Acetazolamide can also cause hepatic difficulties. In patients with hepatic disease, especially cirrhosis, hepatic encephalopathy can occur as a result of hypokalemia and elevations in serum ammonia concentrations during acetazolamide therapy. Disorientation, possibly due to elevated ammonia concentrations, has also been observed in these patients (*Drug Facts and Comparisons*, 2007).

Other Important Metabolic Adverse Effects of Antiepileptic Drugs (al-Rubeaan and Ryan, 1991; *Drug Facts and Comparisons*, 2007)

Metabolic adverse effects of acetazolamide may include hypokalemia, hyperglycemia, glycosuria in patients with diabetes, hyperuricemia, and hyperchloremia.

Metabolic adverse effects of oxcarbazepine may include hyperglycemia, hypocalcemia, hypoglycemia, hypokalemia, and elevated hepatic enzymes.

Phenobarbital, like other barbiturates, can exacerbate porphyria, causing a buildup of porphyrin precursors and enhancing porphyrin synthesis.

Phenytoin can interfere with glucose metabolism. Phenytoin can stimulate glucagon secretion, impair insulin secretion, and cause postbinding defect at the peripheral insulin receptor by affecting $[^{14}C]3,0$-methylglucose transport. Any of these effects could increase serum glucose. Blood sugar should be monitored closely when phenytoin is administered to patients with diabetes mellitus, and this drug is less than desirable for diabetic patients.

Other metabolic adverse effects of valproate may include Fanconi syndrome, hyperglycinemia, and decreased carnitine concentrations.

Rare metabolic adverse effects of zonisamide may include hypoglycemia and hyponatremia.

Lacosamide oral solution contains aspartame, a source of phenylalanine. Patients with phenylketonuria should be advised.

Vigabatrin may increase the amount of amino acids in the urine, possibly leading to a false positive test for certain rare genetic metabolic diseases (e.g., alpha aminoadipic aciduria).

References

al-Rubeaan K, Ryan EA. Phenytoin-induced insulin insensitivity. *Diabetic Medicine*. 1991;8: 968–970.

Asconapé JJ. Some common issues in the use of antiepileptic drugs. *Seminars in Neurology*. 2002;22: 27–39.

Dong X, Leppik IE, White J, Parick J. Hyponatremia from oxcarbazepine and carbam-azepine. *Neurology*. 2005;65: 1967–1978.

Drug Facts and Comparisons. St. Louis: Wolters Kluwer Health/Facts & Comparisons, 2007.

Gankam-Kengne F, Ayers C, Khera A, de Lemos J, Maalouf NM. Mild hyponatremia is associated with an increased risk of death in an ambulatory setting. *Kidney Int*. 2013;83(4): 700–706.

Groeper K, McCann ME. Topiramate and metabolic acidosis: a case series and review of the literature. *Pediatric Anesthesia*. 2005;15: 167–170.

Sachdeo RC, Wasserstein A, Mesenbrink PJ, D'Souza J. Effects of oxcarbazepine on sodium concentration and water handling. *Annals of Neurology*. 2002;51: 613–620.

Sheth RD. Metabolic concerns associated with antiepileptic medications. *Neurology*. 2004;63: S24–S29.

Thakur V, Rupar A, Ramsay DA, Singh R, Fraser DD. Fatal cerebral edema from late-onset ornithine transcarbamylase deficiency in a juvenile male patient receiving valproic acid. *Pediatric Critical Care Medicine*. 2006;7: 273–276.

Verrotti A, Trota D, Morgese G, Chiarelli F. Valproate-induced hyperammonemic encephalopathy. *Metabolic Brain Disease*. 2002;17: 367–373.

Sunovion. http://www.aptiom.com/2014

Eisai. http://www.banzel.com/2014

GSK. http://www.potiga.com/2014

UCB. http://www.vimpat.com/2014

Eisai. http://www.fycompa.com/2014

Lundbeck. http://www.sabril.net/2014

Chapter 15

Antiepileptic Drugs in Patients With Hyperlipidemia

Several reports have already shown that chronic treatment with some antiepileptic drugs (AEDs) influences serum lipid profile. There have been reports of high total cholesterol concentrations in patients receiving carbamazepine, phenytoin, phenobarbital or primidone, high levels of HDL cholesterol in normal subjects receiving phenobarbital and in patients treated with carbamazepine or phenytoin, and high levels of LDL cholesterol in patients treated with carbamazepine and phenobarbital as well as high triglyceride levels in patients receiving carbamazepine, phenobarbital, or phenytoin. An investigation examined lipid levels in adult patients with epilepsy taking phenytoin or carbamazepine who were subsequently switched over to the non-inducing agents lamotrigine or levetiracetam, and found that the change from inducing to noninducing AED led to a decline in total cholesterol averaging 26 mg/dl after only 6 weeks (Mintzer et al., 2009). Influence of valproic acid on serum lipid profiles is controversial (Karikas et al., 2006; Nikolaos et al., 2004; Sommez et al., 2006). Valproate may have adverse long-term metabolic consequences, including obesity, insulin resistance, and the metabolic syndrome, via mechanisms that are presumably distinct from those activated by the inducing drugs (Mintzer et al., 2009).

The effects of AEDs on the serum levels of lipids and lipoproteins could be explained on the basis of the different mechanisms. Carbamazepine, phenytoin, and phenobarbital alter hepatic P-450 microsomal enzyme activity and are metabolized by this same system. This enzyme system catalyzes cholesterol. Thus, carbamazepine, phenytoin, and phenobarbital might compete with cholesterol for utilization of these enzymes and change cholesterol metabolism by altering enzyme levels. The high level of HDL cholesterol could be attributed to the enzyme-inducing properties of carbamazepine, phenytoin, and phenobarbital, which results in an increased hepatic synthesis of apolipoprotein A_1, the major component of HDL cholesterol (Nikolaos et al., 2004). Last, the widely prescribed lipid lowering agents, statins, are metabolized by the cytochrome P-450 complex (Prueksaritanont et al., 1997). Therefore, enzyme-inducing AEDs enhance the clearance of these cholesterol-lowering agents and reduce their effectiveness. For example, co-medication with phenytoin resulted in significant (approximately 50%) reductions in the systemic exposure of atorvastatin (Miller et al., 2008). In vivo studies suggest that eslicarbazepine acetate can induce CYP3A4, decreasing plasma concentrations of drugs that are metabolized by this isoenzyme (e.g., simvastatin). Patients receiving enzyme-inducing AEDs are significantly more likely to require multiple upward dose adjustments of their statin medication (Candrilli et al., 2010).

One should assess the serum lipid profile in patients treated with enzyme-inducing AEDs. In patients with hyperlipidemia it is reasonable to consider switching the patient to a non-inducing AED. A low-cholesterol diet is recommended for patients receiving carbamazepine, phenytoin, phenobarbital, or primidone; oxcarbazepine and topiramate in higher doses (>1200 mg and >200 mg, respectively) are also enzyme inducers, so lipid assessments should be performed as well when enzyme-inducing doses are reached. Treatment with a cholesterol-lowering agent may be indicated as well. Addition of an enzyme-inducing AED may necessitate raising the dose of a cholesterol-lowering agent that has been prescribed.

Recommended Antiepileptic Drugs in Epilepsy Patients With Hyperlipidemia

1. **Generalized epilepsies:** Ethosuximide, lamotrigine, levetiracetam, rufinamide (in patients with Lennox-Gastaut syndrome), zonisamide
2. **Focal epilepsies:** Gabapentin, lacosamide, lamotrigine, levetiracetam, pregabalin, zonisamide

References

Candrilli SD, Manjunath R, Davis KL, Gidal BE. The association between antiepileptic drug and HMG-CoA reductase inhibitor co-medication and cholesterol management in patients with epilepsy. *Epilepsy Res.* 2010; 91(2–3): 260–266.

Karikas GA, Schulpis KH, Bartzeliotou A, et al. Lipids, lipoproteins, apolipoproteins, selected elements and minerals in the serum of children on valproic acid mono-therapy. *Basic and Clinical Pharmacology and Toxicology*, 2006;98: 599–603.

Miller, J. M., Bullman, J. N., Alexander, S., VanLandingham, K. E. A prospective assessment of the effect of phenytoin on the pharmacokinetics of atorvastatin. *Epilepsia.* 2008;49: 444.

Mintzer S, Skidmore CT, Abidin CJ, Morales MC, Chervoneva I, Capuzzi DM, Sperling MR. Effects of antiepileptic drugs on lipids, homocysteine, and C-reactive protein. *Ann Neurol.* 2009;65: 448–456.

Nikolaos T, Stylianos G, Chryssoula N, et al. The effect of long-term antiepileptic treatment on serum cholesterol (TC, HDL, LDL) and triglyceride levels in adult epileptic patients on monotherapy. *Medical Science Monitor.* 2004;10: MT50–MT52.

Prueksaritanont T, Gorham LM, Ma B, et al. In vitro metabolism of simvastatin in humans: identification of metabolizing enzymes and effect of the drug on hepatic P450s. *Drug Metabolism and Disposition.* 1997;25: 1191–1199.

Sonmez FM, Demir E, Orem A, et al. Effect of antiepileptic drugs on plasma lipids, lipoprotein (a), and liver enzymes. *Journal of Child Neurology*. 2006;21: 70–74.

Sunovion. http://www.aptiom.com/2014

Eisai. http://www.banzel.com/2014

GSK. http://www.potiga.com/2014

UCB. http://www.vimpat.com/2014

Eisai. http://www.fycompa.com/2014

Lundbeck. http://www.sabril.net/2014

Chapter 16

Antiepileptic Drugs in Patients With Diabetes Mellitus

Selection of the appropriate antiepileptic therapy should be guided by the recognition that some patients have multiple comorbidities and receive multiple medications. Antiepileptic drugs (AEDs) may have various adverse or beneficial effects in patients with diabetes mellitus (DM).

Acetazolamide

Acetazolamide has rarely caused severe metabolic acidosis in patients with diabetes mellitus (Zaidi & Kinnear, 2004). Diabetic patients should be monitored for a loss of blood glucose control and electrolyte disturbances.

Carbamazepine

Carbamazepine is US Food and Drug Administration approved for trigeminal neuralgia and may also help painful diabetic neuropathy (Maizels & McCarberg, 2005; Vinik, 2005).

Ezogabine

Ezogabine was associated with dose-related weight gain. It is not an optimal drug for patients with DM.

Perampanel

Perampanel was associated with weight gain. It is not an optimal drug for patients with DM.

Phenytoin

Phenytoin may impair insulin release and cause insulin insensitivity and hyperglycemia, so this drug should be avoided in patients with diabetes. These adverse effects may cause temporary loss of glycemic control in diabetic patients. Close observation is necessary to maintain adequate glycemic control in patients with diabetes mellitus (al-Rubeaan & Rayan, 1991).

Gabapentin

Gabapentin is useful for postherpetic neuralgia and may also be appropriate for painful diabetic neuropathy (Maizels & McCarberg, 2005; Vinik, 2005). However, it causes weight gain in some patients and is therefore suboptimal as a first-line choice for epilepsy treatment. Studies have reported fluctuations in blood sugar levels, and this should be considered in diabetic patients.

Lamotrigine

Lamotrigine does not pose problems with regard to diabetes and may be appropriate for painful diabetic neuropathy (Vinik, 2005).

Levetiracetam

Levetiracetam induced an antihyperalgesic effect in two models of human neuropathic pain, suggesting a therapeutic potential in neuropathic pain patients (Ardid et al., 2003). Human studies are scarce and conflicting.

Pregabalin

Pregabalin is efficacious for painful diabetic neuropathy (Maizels & McCarberg, 2005; Vinik, 2005). Pregabalin treatment did not appear to be associated with loss of glycemic control. However, as the thiazolidinedione class of antidiabetic drugs can cause weight gain and fluid retention, possibly exacerbating diabetes or leading to heart failure, it should not be considered a first-line drug for primary treatment of seizure disorders (Laustsen et al., 2006). Pregabalin has the potential to cause an increase in appetite (in 5% of patients) and might cause weight gain (in 4%–12%).

Topiramate

Topiramate may occasionally help the pain of diabetic neuropathy (Vinik, 2005). In addition, topiramate treatment of overweight diabetic patients can result in significant weight reduction and loss of body fat, leading to improvement in the glycemic control (Eliasson et al., 2007).

Valproate

Valproate is associated with weight gain, alteration of adipocytokine homeostasis, insulin resistance and non-alcoholic fatty liver disease (Rauchenzauner et al., 2013). Therefore, it is not an optimal drug for patients with DM.

Vigabatrin

Vigabatrin causes weight gain in adult and pediatric patients. Weight gain is not related to the occurrence of edema. Besides, it may cause symptoms of peripheral neuropathy. Therefore, it is not an optimal drug for patients with DM.

Zonisamide

Zonisamide may lead to weight loss in some individuals, leading to improvement in glycemic control.

Recommended Antiepileptic Drugs in Epilepsy Patients With Diabetes Mellitus

1. **Generalized epilepsies:** Lamotrigine, levetiracetam, topiramate, zonisamide
2. **Focal epilepsies:** Levetiracetam, carbamazepine, lamotrigine, topiramate, zonisamide. If neuropathy is present, consider gabapentin or pregabalin, although lamotrigine, carbamazepine, and topiramate may offer benefit as well.

Note: Carbamazepine, pregabalin, and gabapentin may cause weight gain, which is not desirable in diabetic patients. In contrast, topiramate and zonisamide may cause weight loss, which may be favorable in diabetic patients (Biton, 2006).

References

al-Rubeaan K, Rayan EA. Phenytoin-induced insulin insensitivity. *Diabetic Medicine*. 1991;8: 968–970.

Ardid D, Lamberty Y, Alloui A, Coudore-Civiale MA, Klitgaard H, Eschalier A. Antihyperalgesic effect of levetiracetam in neuropathic pain models in rats. *Eur J Pharmacol*. 2003;473(1): 27–33.

Biton V. Weight change and antiepileptic drugs. *The Neurologist*. 2006;10: 163–167.

Eliasson B, Gudbjornsdottir S, Cederholm J, Liang Y, Vercruysse F, Smith U. Weight loss and metabolic effects of topiramate in overweight and obese type 2 diabetic patients: randomized double-blind placebo-controlled trial. *International Journal of Obesity*. 2007;31: 1140–1147.

Laustsen G, Gilbert M, Wimett L. A look back at the influential drug approvals of 2005. *Nurse Practitioner*. 2006;31: 29–36.

Maizels M, McCarberg B. Antidepressants and antiepileptic drugs for chronic non-cancer pain. *American Family Physician*. 2005;71: 483–490.

Rauchenzauner M, Laimer M, Wiedmann M, et al. The novel insulin resistance parameters RBP4 and GLP-1 in patients treated with valproic acid: just a side-step? *Epilepsy Res*. 2013;104(3): 285–288.

Vinik A. Clinical review: use of antiepileptic drugs in the treatment of chronic painful diabetic neuropathy. *Journal of Clinical Endocrinology and Metabolism*. 2005;90: 4936–4945.

Zaidi FH, Kinnear PE. Acetazolamide, alternate carbonic anhydrase inhibitors and hypoglycaemic agents: comparing enzymatic with diuresis induced metabolic acidosis following intraocular surgery in diabetes. *British Journal of Ophthalmology*. 2004;88: 714–715.

Sunovion. http://www.aptiom.com/2014

Eisai. http://www.banzel.com/2014

GSK. http://www.potiga.com/2014

UCB. http://www.vimpat.com/2014

Eisai. http://www.fycompa.com/2014

Lundbeck. http://www.sabril.net/2014

Chapter 17

Antiepileptic Drugs in Patients With Cardiovascular Disorders

Selection of the appropriate antiepileptic therapy should be guided by the recognition that some patients have multiple comorbidities and receive multiple medications. Antiepileptic drugs (AEDs) may have adverse effects on cardiovascular system. In addition, patients with cardiovascular disorders are usually on antihypertensive, anticoagulant, or cardiac drugs, which may have significant interactions with AEDs.

A number of serologic markers relevant to cardiovascular risk have been found to be affected by the CYP450-inducing AEDs. These include cholesterol and specific atherogenic lipid fractions, lipoprotein(a), CRP, and homocysteine. These alterations suggest that enzyme-inducing AEDs might produce elevations in cardiovascular risk, a notion reinforced by the epidemiologic data. Monitoring vascular risk factors in patients receiving CYP450-inducing AEDs may be beneficial. Besides, newer non-enzyme-inducing AEDs such as lacosamide, lamotrigine, and levetiracetam may be safer when prescribed to patients with a high risk of developing atherosclerosis, as indicated by family history of occlusive vascular disease or genetic disorders that lead to hyperhomocysteinemia, but whether the newer AEDs are clearly beneficial in this context remains to be evaluated (Jakubus et al., 2009; Mintzer 2010; Svalheim et al., 2010).

The major class of drug-drug interaction is between AEDs that induce or inhibit the cytochrome P-450 enzyme system and cardiovascular medications that are metabolized by these enzymes. Therefore, it is best to avoid enzyme-altering AEDs if possible. Some cardiovascular drugs inhibit these hepatic enzymes and so may produce AED side effects and toxicity. Similarly, AEDs that are highly protein bound have interactions with cardiovascular drugs that bind to serum proteins, and similar cautions apply. Specific drug-disease and drug-drug interactions of AEDs with cardiovascular system and drugs are listed below (Dhatt et al., 1979; Kenneback et al., 1991; Laine et al., 2000; Parrish et al., 2006; *Drug Facts and Comparisons*, 2007; Drugs' websites).

Acetazolamide

Acetazolamide can cause hypokalemia. Therefore, patients receiving acetazolamide concurrently with cardiac glycosides are at an increased risk for cardiac toxicity if hypokalemia develops during treatment.

Benzodiazepines

CYP3A4 inhibitors may reduce the metabolism of clonazepam and increase the probability for benzodiazepine toxicity. Examples of CYP3A4 inhibitors include amiodarone, diltiazem, nicardipine, and verapamil. Monitor patients who receive concurrent therapy.

Carbamazepine

Cardiovascular adverse effects that can develop during carbamazepine therapy include atrioventricular block, cardiac arrhythmias or arrhythmia exacerbation, congestive heart failure, edema, aggravation of hypertension, hypotension, syncope, thrombophlebitis, and thromboembolism. Some cardiovascular complications have resulted in death. However, severe cardiac complications generally occur only when very high doses (>60 g) have been ingested. Carbamazepine should be used with caution in any patient with cardiac disease, such as cardiac arrhythmias, congestive heart failure, or coronary artery disease. The drug should not be used in patients with atrioventricular block or other conduction abnormalities (bundle-branch block) (Kenneback et al., 1991). Carbamazepine is an enzyme-inducing AED and may affect serologic markers that are relevant to cardiovascular risk.

Carbamazepine is metabolized by the hepatic isoenzyme CYP3A4. Many drugs (e.g., diltiazem and verapamil) are known to inhibit CYP3A4 and may decrease carbamazepine metabolism, thereby increasing carbamazepine plasma concentrations. Serum carbamazepine concentrations should be monitored closely if any of these agents are added during carbamazepine therapy. It may be necessary to reduce the dose of carbamazepine in this situation. Conversely, carbamazepine may induce the hepatic metabolism of calcium channel blockers, which reduces the levels of these drugs. Carbamazepine is also protein bound, and its concentration may be altered by or alter that of other protein-bound drugs.

Carbamazepine induces the metabolism of warfarin and dicumarol requiring the dosage of anticoagulants to be increased over several weeks after initiating carbamazepine therapy. If carbamazepine is discontinued, dosage reductions of warfarin or dicumarol are usually necessary. Patients on oral anticoagulation should be monitored closely for changes in the INR when carbamazepine is added or discontinued from a patient's drug therapy regimen (Parrish et al., 2006).

Eslicarbazepine Acetate

Compared to placebo, eslicarbazepine acetate use was associated with slightly higher frequencies of increases in total cholesterol, triglycerides, and LDL. Patients receiving warfarin should be monitored to maintain INR.

Ezogabine

Ezogabine might cause QT prolongation. The QT interval should be monitored when ezogabine is prescribed with medicines known to increase QT interval and in patients with known prolonged QT interval, congestive heart failure, ventricular hypertrophy, hypokalemia, or hypomagnesemia.

Data from an in vitro study showed that the N-acetyl metabolite of ezogabine inhibited P-glycoprotein mediated transport of digoxin in a concentration-dependent manner. Administration of ezogabine at therapeutic doses may increase digoxin serum concentrations. Serum levels of digoxin should be monitored.

Gabapentin

Hypertension has been reported with gabapentin therapy, occurring at an incidence greater than 1%.

The combination of propranolol and gabapentin may induce dystonia via a pharmacodynamic interaction.

Lacosamide

Dose-dependent prolongations in PR interval with lacosamide have been observed. First-degree atrioventricular (AV) block, second degree, and complete AV blocks have been reported. Lacosamide should be used with caution in patients with known conduction problems (e.g., marked first-degree AV block, second-degree or higher AV block, and sick sinus syndrome without pacemaker), sodium channelopathies (e.g., Brugada Syndrome), on concomitant medications that prolong PR interval, or with severe cardiac disease such as myocardial ischemia or heart failure, or structural heart disease. In such patients, obtaining an ECG before beginning lacosamide, and after lacosamide is titrated to steady-state, is recommended. Lacosamide administration may predispose the patient to atrial arrhythmias (atrial fibrillation or flutter), especially in those with diabetic neuropathy and/or cardiovascular disease. Lacosamide may rarely cause palpitation, bradycardia, or syncope.

Oxcarbazepine

Sinus bradycardia, sinus tachycardia, heart failure, hypertension, orthostatic hypotension, palpitations, and syncope have been reported with oxcarbazepine. However, the role of oxcarbazepine in their causation cannot be reliably determined. Hepatic enzyme inhibitors may delay conversion of oxcarbazepine to its active metabolite.

Phenobarbital/Primidone

Phenobarbital and primidone are enzyme-inducing AEDs and may affect serologic markers that are relevant to cardiovascular risk.

A serious drug interaction can occur between barbiturates and warfarin. All barbiturates are hepatic enzyme inducers, and the clinical effects of warfarin can be compromised if a barbiturate is added. More importantly, discontinuation of a barbiturate during warfarin therapy may lead to fatal bleeding. Warfarin doses would require readjustment if a barbiturate is added or discontinued during warfarin therapy (Laine et al., 2000).

Barbiturates can enhance the hepatic metabolism of β-blockers that are significantly metabolized by the liver (betaxolol, labetalol, metoprolol, pindolol, propranolol, and timolol). Patient should be monitored for loss of β-blockade.

Barbiturates may interact with cardiac glycosides. Barbiturates can accelerate the metabolism of digoxin, decreasing digoxin serum concentrations.

Concurrent use of phenobarbital with some antihypertensive agents may lead to excessive hypotension. In addition, barbiturates have been shown to enhance the hepatic clearance of the calcium channel blockers (e.g., diltiazem, nifedipine, and verapamil). When selecting alternative therapy to a barbiturate is not possible, patients should be monitored for the desired cardiovascular effects of these drugs.

Parenteral administration of barbiturates should be given cautiously to patients with hypertension, hypotension, cardiac disease, or other hemodynamically unstable conditions (i.e., heart failure, shock).

Phenytoin

Phenytoin should be used with caution in patients with cardiac disease (e.g., cardiac arrhythmias, congestive heart failure, or coronary artery disease). The drug should not be used in patients with cardiac conduction abnormalities (e.g., bundle-branch block) (Dhatt et al., 1979). Phenytoin is an enzyme-inducing AED and may affect serologic markers that are relevant to cardiovascular risk.

Parenteral phenytoin should be used with caution in patients with cardiac disease, because it can cause atrial and ventricular conduction depression, hypotension, ventricular fibrillation, and reduced cardiac output. The rate of intravenous administration of phenytoin is important (i.e., maximum infusion rate is 50 mg/min in adults).

The interaction between warfarin and phenytoin is complex. An immediate interaction may occur, as phenytoin can displace warfarin from its protein-binding sites, causing rapid increases in the INR. After prolonged administration, phenytoin may reduce the effectiveness of warfarin by inducing the hepatic metabolism of warfarin. Warfarin dosage adjustments may be necessary if phenytoin is added. Competitive inhibition may also occur since phenytoin and warfarin are both substrates for cytochrome P-450 2C9. Warfarin may alter phenytoin serum concentrations as well. Phenytoin also may deplete vitamin K–dependent clotting factors after prolonged therapy. Similar interactions may occur between phenytoin or fosphenytoin and dicumarol. Oral anticoagulant dosage adjustments may also be necessary on discontinuation of phenytoin or fosphenytoin therapy.

Phenytoin clearance can be decreased by drugs that inhibit hepatic microsomal enzymes, particularly those drugs that significantly inhibit the cytochrome P-450 2C subset of isoenzymes (e.g., amiodarone and ticlopidine). Phenytoin or fosphenytoin dosage adjustments may be necessary in patients who receive any of these drugs concurrently. Monitor the patient for signs of phenytoin toxicity.

Hydantoin anticonvulsants induce hepatic microsomal enzymes and may increase the metabolism of cardiac glycosides, atorvastatin, simvastatin, and calcium channel blockers.

Pregabalin

Pregabalin should be used cautiously in patients with severe heart failure. Dose-related weight gain and peripheral edema have been noted with pregabalin.

Rufinamide

ECG studies demonstrated shortening of the QT interval with rufinamide treatment. However, there was no signal for drug-induced sudden death or ventricular arrhythmias. The degree of QT shortening induced by rufinamide is without any known clinical risk. Familial Short QT syndrome is associated with an increased risk of sudden death and ventricular arrhythmias, particularly ventricular fibrillation. Patients with Familial Short QT syndrome should not be treated with rufinamide. Caution should be used when administering rufinamide with other drugs that shorten the QT interval.

Topiramate

Hypertension and bradycardia are among infrequent adverse effects of topiramate. Although the clinical relevance has not been determined, the clinician should be aware that serum digoxin concentrations may be decreased when digoxin and topiramate are used concomitantly.

Valproic Acid

Cardiovascular side effects of valproate include hypertension, palpitation, tachycardia, and bradycardia.

Concurrent administration of highly protein-bound agents such as valproate may displace warfarin from its binding sites, leading to increased anticoagulation. Monitor INR closely when valproate therapy is introduced or stopped.

Zonisamide

Cardiovascular adverse effects have been infrequently reported with zonisamide therapy. These adverse effects included hypertension, hypotension, palpitation, sinus bradycardia, sinus tachycardia, syncope, thrombophlebitis, and vascular insufficiency. Rare cardiovascular adverse reactions include atrial fibrillation, heart failure, pulmonary embolus, and ventricular extrasystole.

Zonisamide is metabolized by hepatic CYP3A4. Inhibitors including diltiazem, nicardipine, ranolazine, and verapamil can increase the systemic exposure of zonisamide by decreasing the metabolism of the drug.

Recommended Antiepileptic Drugs in Epilepsy Patients With Cardiovascular Disorders

1. **Generalized epilepsies:** Ethosuximide, lamotrigine, levetiracetam
2. **Focal epilepsies:** Lamotrigine, levetiracetam, oxcarbazepine, perampanel.

References

Dhatt MS, Gomes JA, Reddy CP, Akhtar M, Caracta AR, Lau SH, Damato AN. Effects of phenytoin on refractoriness and conduction in the human heart. *Journal of Cardiovascular Pharmacology.* 1979;1: 3–18.

Drug Facts and Comparisons. St. Louis: Wolters Kluwer Health/Facts & Comparisons, St Louis, 2007.

Jakubus T, Michalska-Jakubus M, Lukawski K, Janowska A, Czuczwar SJ. Atherosclerotic risk among children taking antiepileptic drugs. *Pharmacol Rep.* 2009;61(3): 411–423.

Kenneback G, Bergfeldt L, Vallin H, Tomson T, Edhag O. Electrophysiologic effects and clinical hazards of carbamazepine treatment for neurologic disorders in patients with abnormalities of the cardiac conduction system. *American Heart Journal.* 1991;121: 1421–1429.

Laine K, Forsstrom J, Gronroos P, Irjala K, Kailajarvi M, Scheinin M. Frequency and clinical outcome of potentially harmful drug metabolic interactions in patients hospitalized on internal and pulmonary medicine wards: focus on warfarin and cisapride. *Therapeutic Drug Monitoring.* 2000;22: 503–509.

Mintzer S. Metabolic consequences of antiepileptic drugs. *Curr Opin Neurol.* 2010;23: 164–169.

Parrish RH, Pazdur DE, O'Donnell PJ. Effect of carbamazepine initiation and discontinuation on antithrombotic control in a patient receiving warfarin: case report and review of the literature. *Pharmacotherapy.* 2006;26: 1650–1653.

Svalheim S, Luef G, Rauchenzauner M, Mørkrid L, Gjerstad L, Taubøll E. Cardiovascular risk factors in epilepsy patients taking levetiracetam, carbamazepine or lamotrigine. Acta *Neurol Scand.* 2010;122 (Suppl. 190): 30–33.

Sunovion. http://www.aptiom.com/2014
Eisai. http://www.banzel.com/2014
GSK. http://www.potiga.com/2014
UCB. http://www.vimpat.com/2014
Eisai. http://www.fycompa.com/2014
Lundbeck. http://www.sabril.net/2014

Chapter 18

Antiepileptic Drugs in Patients With Hematological Disorders

Many antiepileptic drugs (AEDs) are associated with hematological toxicity (Levy et al., 2002; *Drug Facts and Comparisons*, 2007; Verrotti et al., 2014). A wide spectrum of hematological abnormalities can be seen after prescribing an AED, ranging from mild thrombocytopenia or neutropenia to anemia, red cell aplasia, or even bone marrow failure. The magnitude of the problem is illustrated by the fact that at least one hematological abnormality was noted in 33% of patients taking valproate in one study (May and Sunder, 1993). Transient leukopenia has been reported in 12% of patients taking carbamazepine (Asadi-Pooya & Ghetmiri, 2006), while persistent leukopenia occurs in 2% of patients (Verrotti et al., 2014). Phenytoin produces similar rates of leukopenia. These abnormalities are usually inconsequential, but as noted, serious life-threatening illnesses may be provoked by AED therapy. Fortunately, potentially fatal hematological disorders are rare; for example, aplastic anemia has an incidence of only a few cases per million per year. Nonetheless, knowledge of the hematological adverse effects of these drugs is crucial when selecting AEDs in patients with epilepsy. For example, cytochrome P-450 enzymes are hemoproteins and play an important role in drug metabolism, particularly in the liver. As a result of enzyme induction, more of these hemoproteins are synthesized, which in turn induces heme synthesis. Increased heme synthesis then leads to accelerated porphyrin production and may result in an acute attack of porphyria. Many drugs that have hepatic metabolism are labeled as porphyrinogenic and are potentially dangerous in patients with porphyria and therefore should be avoided. AEDs such as levetiracetam, perampanel, gabapentin, and pregabalin are preferred in epilepsy patients with porphyria due to their negligible hepatic metabolism.

Whether patients with underlying primary hematological disorders are at greater risk for adverse effects when prescribed AEDs is uncertain. Due to the relatively common provocation of hematological abnormalities by some drugs, however, it seems prudent to avoid their use in patients who have less functional reserve. This chapter will review hematological effects known to be associated with the use of AEDs.

Acetazolamide

Acetazolamide rarely induces bone marrow suppression, but cases of fatal aplastic anemia and thrombocytopenia have been reported. Patients with hematological disease should have periodic hematological evaluations, probably no more often than warranted for their clinical condition, however.

Benzodiazepines

Significant hematological adverse effects, such as thrombocytopenia, leucopenia, agranulocytosis, and pancytopenia are quite rare (Verrotti et al., 2014).

Carbamazepine

Carbamazepine should be used with caution in patients with blood dyscrasias caused by drugs or other hematological diseases. The overall incidence of severe hematological side effects of carbamazepine is estimated to be 1:38,000 to 1:10,800 in various studies. These serious side effects include aplastic anemia, agranulocytosis, and pancytopenia. Carbamazepine has also been associated with thrombocytopenia. Mild anemia has been reported in less than 5% of the patients taking carbamazepine. The risk of developing these adverse reactions is 5–8 times greater in patients treated with carbamazepine than in the general population. If pretreatment baseline complete blood counts are abnormal, periodic monitoring of blood counts is advisable; no objective data exist to advise a correct monitoring regimen. The authors would check the blood count 1 month or so after initiating therapy and then every few months for the first year. And then, the blood count would be checked yearly in these patients with abnormal pretreatment baseline complete blood counts, assuming no problems are detected. If neutropenia or thrombocytopenia develops, the patient should be closely monitored. Discontinuation of carbamazepine should be considered if the total leukocyte (white blood cell [WBC]) count falls below 2000/mL, the neutrophil (polymorphonuclear cell [PMN]) count falls below 1000/mL, the erythrocyte count falls below 3.5×10^6/mL, the platelet count falls below 80,000/mL, or the hemoglobin concentration falls below 11 g/dL. In most cases, leukopenia, thrombocytopenia, and other adverse effects are usually milder and transient, and cessation is rarely necessary (Rush & Beran, 1984; Joffe et al., 1985; Olcay et al., 1995; Tohen et al., 1995; Verrotti et al., 2014). These guidelines are applicable for all AEDs. Folate supplementation may prevent carbamazepine-induced leucopenia or anemia (Asadi-Pooya & Ghetmiri, 2006). Because carbamazepine may exacerbate porphyria, this drug should be avoided in that disease.

Eslicarbazepine Acetate

Hematological adverse events are quite rare. Compared to placebo, eslicarbazepine acetate use was associated with slightly higher frequencies of anemia.

Ethosuximide

Ethosuximide should be used with caution in patients with bone marrow suppression or any hematological disease. Blood dyscrasias including leukopenia, eosinophilia, agranulocytosis, aplastic anemia, and pancytopenia have been reported to be associated with ethosuximide treatment. Discontinue the drug if counts fall below the parameters mentioned in the preceding paragraph (see Carbamazepine).

Ezogabine

Hematological adverse events are quite rare. Leukopenia, neutropenia, and thrombocytopenia have been reported rarely.

Felbamate

Treatment with felbamate has been associated with an increase in the incidence of aplastic anemia. The incidence of aplastic anemia has been reported to be 27–209 per million users for those receiving felbamate (most probable value of 127 per million users) versus about 2–2.5 per million persons in the general population (Kaufman et al., 1997). The aplastic anemia population risk for felbamate treatment is 20 times greater than that for carbamazepine (Kaufman et al., 1997). Therefore, felbamate should only be used in patients with severe epilepsy posing significant risk of injury and harm that is unresponsive to other AEDs. It is not certain whether the risk of developing aplastic anemia changes with the duration of treatment or dose of felbamate, but nearly all reported cases have occurred within the first year of treatment. Routine blood testing cannot reliably predict the incidence of aplastic anemia but allows the detection of the hematological changes early in their course. Felbamate should be discontinued if any evidence of bone marrow suppression occurs.

Other infrequent hematological adverse effects of felbamate include lymphadenopathy, leukocytosis, and thrombocytopenia. Antinuclear factor test–positive, qualitative platelet disorder, and agranulocytosis have been rarely reported.

Gabapentin

Hematological adverse events are quite rare. The reported incidence of leukopenia with gabapentin treatment is about 1.1%, and it is usually mild. The hematological adverse effect more often reported is purpura or bruising from physical trauma. Reports of thrombocytopenia, anemia, and lymphadenopathy have been rare.

Lacosamide

Hematological adverse events are quite rare. Rarely, agranulocytosis, neutropenia and anemia have been reported.

Lamotrigine

Hematological adverse effects observed during lamotrigine therapy include anemia, eosinophilia, leukopenia, thrombocytopenia, and disseminated intravascular coagulation. These adverse reactions are rare. Although lamotrigine has weak antifolate activity, no clinically significant alterations in serum or erythrocyte folate concentrations have been identified with lamotrigine therapy (Gidal et al., 2005).

Levetiracetam

Leukopenia and neutropenia have been infrequently reported in adults and children receiving levetiracetam. Most of these reactions are transient, and usually there is no need for drug discontinuation. Mild anemia has also been reported in adults. Pancytopenia has been reported in post-marketing reports; however, no causal relationship has been established. Levetiracetam seems to inhibit thromboxane-dependent platelet activation and aggregation. It is suggested that caution should be exercised when this drug is used concomitantly with antithrombotic drugs, especially with antiplatelet agents such as clopidogrel, because of an expected additive effect (Verrotti et al., 2014).

Oxcarbazepine

Leukopenia and thrombocytopenia have been reported with oxcarbazepine treatment but are rare.

Perampanel

Hematological adverse events are quite rare.

Phenobarbital

Megaloblastic anemia, leukopenia, agranulocytosis, and thrombocytopenia have been reported with phenobarbital treatment. Megaloblastic anemia may respond to folate supplementation, allowing continued phenobarbital therapy. Because phenobarbital may exacerbate porphyria, this drug should be avoided in that disease.

Phenytoin

Phenytoin should be used with caution in patients with blood dyscrasias caused by drugs or other hematological diseases. Phenytoin can cause hematological adverse effects including thrombocytopenia, leukopenia, neutropenia, agranulocytosis, pancytopenia, macrocytosis, and megaloblastic anemia. However, serious blood dyscrasias are rare in patients taking phenytoin (Blackburn et al., 1998). Monitoring guidelines are similar to those for carbamazepine. Although macrocytosis and megaloblastic anemia usually respond to therapy with folate, they are uncommon, and folate need not be administered routinely to patients receiving phenytoin. Folate has potential detrimental effects on phenytoin plasma levels and efficacy that may cause seizure exacerbation (Steinweg & Bentley, 2005).

Because phenytoin may exacerbate porphyria, this drug should be avoided in that disease. Phenytoin may rarely cause hemolysis as an adverse reaction; use with caution in patients with hemolytic anemia. Methemoglobinemia is rare with normal therapeutic doses of phenytoin; however, this adverse effect has occasionally been reported, especially in the setting of overdose or in patients with methemoglobin reductase deficiency.

There are some reports about a relationship between phenytoin and the development of lymphadenopathy (local or generalized) including benign lymph node hyperplasia, pseudolymphoma, lymphoma, and Hodgkin's disease. Although a cause-and-effect relationship has not been established, the occurrence of lymphadenopathy requires investigation, and phenytoin should be stopped.

Pregabalin

Pregabalin treatment has been associated with thrombocytopenia, although this is rare.

Rufinamide

Anemia has been reported with rufinamide use. Other hematological adverse effects are infrequent and include lymphadenopathy, leucopenia, neutropenia, and thrombocytopenia.

Topiramate

Epistaxis has been reported to occur in 1%–4% of patients with topiramate treatment. Topiramate may modulate voltage-gated L-type calcium ion channels located on vascular smooth muscle and platelets. Bleeding tendency associated with topiramate may be more pronounced in patients receiving concomitant antiplatelet therapy. Hematological complications (e.g., anemia) are rare.

Valproate

Thrombocytopenia (dose-dependent), inhibition of the secondary phase of platelet aggregation, and abnormal coagulation parameters (e.g., low fibrinogen) have been reported with valproate treatment. A decrease in platelet count is the most common hematological effect of valproate. While the reported incidence varies from 5% to 60%, this is usually transient, and sustained thrombocytopenia is uncommon in our experience. Clinically significant bleeding is uncommon because the thrombocytopenia is usually not severe. Thrombocytopenia usually develops after several months of high valproate levels (>100 µg/mL), but resolves within a few days after dose reduction (Suchitra & James, 2000; Gerstner et al., 2006). Platelet counts are recommended before initiating valproic acid therapy and at periodic intervals if clinical signs appear. If an increased bleeding tendency is observed before surgical procedures, it is recommended to assess platelet count, thrombelastography, PT, aPTT, TT, fibrinogen, vWF, and factor XIII. Hemorrhages, hematomas, petechiae, bruising, and prolonged bleeding time are indications for dosage reduction or withdrawal of therapy (Verrotti et al., 2014).

Mild leukopenia, neutropenia, bone marrow suppression, lymphadenopathy, and exacerbation of acute intermittent porphyria have been reported with valproic acid therapy (Suchitra & James, 2000). Any evidence of hemorrhage, bruising, hematomas, petechiae, or a disorder of hemostasis or coagulation (e.g., prolonged bleeding time) is an indication for reduction of the dosage or withdrawal of therapy.

Vigabatrin

Anemia has been reported with vigabatrin use. Other hematological adverse events are quite rare.

Zonisamide

Ecchymosis is a hematological adverse reaction occasionally associated with zonisamide therapy. Also, anemia, immunodeficiency, leukopenia, and lymphadenopathy have rarely been reported. Rare adverse reactions include microcytic anemia, petechiae, and thrombocytopenia.

Recommended Antiepileptic Drugs in Epilepsy Patients With Bone Marrow Suppression or Hematological Disorders

1. **Generalized epilepsies:** Benzodiazepines, lamotrigine, levetiracetam
2. **Focal epilepsies:** Eslicarbazepine acetate, gabapentin, lacosamide, lamotrigine, levetiracetam, oxcarbazepine, perampanel

References

Asadi-Pooya AA, Ghetmiri E. Folic acid supplementation reduces the development of some blood cell abnormalities in children receiving carbamazepine. *Epilepsy and Behavior*. 2006;8: 228–231.

Blackburn SC, Oliart AD, Garcia Rodriguez LA. Antiepileptics and blood dyscrasias: a cohort study. *Pharmacotherapy*. 1998;18: 1277–1283.

Drug Facts and Comparisons. St. Louis: Wolters Kluwer Health/Facts & Comparisons, 2007.

Gerstner T, Teich M, Bell N, Longin E, Dempfle CE, Brand J, Konig S. Valproate-associated coagulopathies are frequent and variable in children. *Epilepsia*. 2006;47: 1136–1143.

Gidal BE, Tamura T, Hammer A, Vuong A. Blood homocysteine, folate and vitamin B-12 concentrations in patients with epilepsy receiving lamotrigine or sodium valproate for initial monotherapy. *Epilepsy Research*. 2005;64: 161–166.

Joffe RT, Post RM, Roy-Byrne PP, et al. Hematological effects of carbamazepine in patients with affective illness. *American Journal of Psychiatry*. 1985;142: 1196–1199.

Kaufman DW, Kelly JP, Anderson T, et al. Evaluation of case reports of aplastic anemia among patients treated with felbamate. *Epilepsia*. 1997;38: 1265–1269.

Levy RH, Mattson RH, Meldrum BS, Perucca E. *Antiepileptic Drugs*, 5th ed. Philadelphia: Lippincott Williams & Wilkins, 2002.

May R, Sunder TR. Hematologic manifestations of long-term valproate therapy. *Epilepsia*. 1993;34: 1098–1101.

Olcay L, Pekcan S, Yalnizoglu D, et al. Fatal agranulocytosis developed in the course of carbamazepine therapy. *Turkish Journal of Pediatrics*. 1995;37: 73–77.

Rush JA, Beran RG. Leucopenia as an adverse reaction to carbamazepine therapy. *Medical Journal of Australia*. 1984;140: 426–428.

Steinweg DL, Bentley ML. Seizures following reduction in phenytoin level after orally administered folic acid. *Neurology*. 2005;64: 1982.

Suchitra A, James B. Hematologic toxicity of sodium valproate. *Journal of Pediatric Hematology*. 2000;22: 62–65.

Tohen M, Castillo PHJ, Baldessarini RJ, et al. Blood dyscrasias with carbamazepine and valproate: a pharmacoepidemiological study of 2228 patients at risk. *Am J Psychiatry*. 1995;152: 413–418.

Verrotti A, Scaparrotta A, Grosso S, Chiarelli F, Coppola G. Anticonvulsant drugs and hematological disease. *Neurol Sci* 2014;35(7): 983–993.

Sunovion. http://www.aptiom.com/2014

Eisai. http://www.banzel.com/2014

GSK. http://www.potiga.com/2014

UCB. http://www.vimpat.com/2014

Eisai. http://www.fycompa.com/2014

Lundbeck. http://www.sabril.net/2014

Chapter 19

Antiepileptic Drugs in Patients on Chemotherapy or Immunosuppressive Therapy

Patients with cancer are at high risk for drug-drug interactions, because anticancer drugs not only possess a complex pharmacologic profile but also may possess a narrow therapeutic index and a steep dose toxicity curve. Antiepileptic drugs (AEDs) are indicated in patients with cancer who present with epilepsy. Chemotherapeutic agents may lose effectiveness when enzyme-inducing AEDs are prescribed because many chemotherapeutic agents are also metabolized by the cytochrome P-450 enzyme system (Box 19.1). These AEDs include phenobarbital, primidone, phenytoin, and carbamazepine, as well as oxcarbazepine and topiramate in higher doses. On the other hand, enzyme-inhibiting AEDs, such as valproic acid, may amplify hematologic and other toxicities of chemotherapeutic agents (e.g., nitrosoureas or etoposide). It is therefore advisable to use AEDs that do not interfere with the cytochrome P-450 enzyme complex and have low protein binding, when treating patients who require chemotherapy (Patsalos et al., 2002; Oberndorfer et al., 2005; Vecht and van Breemen, 2006; Yap et al., 2008; Perucca 2013).

Similar recommendations are applicable for patients on immunosuppressive therapy (e.g., transplant patients). For example, carbamazepine, oxcarbazepine, phenobarbital, and phenytoin reduce cyclosporine, tacrolimus, and corticosteroid blood levels. However, there are other considerations in transplant patients (Chabolla & Wszolek, 2006):

1. Toxicity from AEDs is more common in patients with coexisting hepatic or renal dysfunction.
2. Drugs such as phenytoin, carbamazepine, and valproate are heavily protein bound; only unbound or free drug is pharmacologically active. Although free drug concentration can be estimated from total concentration, for strongly bound drugs, prediction of free level is not always possible. Conditions like uremia, liver disease, and hypoalbuminemia, which are commonly observed in transplant patients, can lead to significant increases in free drug, resulting in drug toxicity even if the concentration of total drug is within therapeutic range (Chabolla & Wszolek, 2006; Dasgupta, 2007).

> ### Box 19.1 *Panel:* Commonly used anticancer drugs negatively affected by co-medication with enzyme-inducing antiepileptic drugs
>
> **Alkylating Agents**
>
> Carmustine, lomustine, nimustine, fotemustine (nitrosoureas); thiotepa; cyclophosphamide; ifosfamide
>
> **Mitotic Inhibitors**
>
> Vincristine, vinorelbine (vinca-alcaloids); paclitaxel; docetaxel
>
> **Topoisomerase Inhibitors/DNA-damaging agents**
>
> Irinotecan, topotecan, etoposide, doxorubicin
>
> **Antimetabolites**
>
> Methotrexate pemetrexed
>
> **Signal Transduction Inhibitors**
>
> Imatinib, erlotinib, gefinitib, sorafenib, temsirolimus, everolimus, vemurafenib
>
> **Proteasome Inhibitors**
>
> Bortezomib
>
> Adapted from: Weller M, Stupp R, Wick W. Epilepsy meets cancer: when, why, and what to do about it? *Lancet Oncol* 2012;13(9): e375–e382.

3. Hypersensitivity can occur with agents such as carbamazepine, oxcarbazepine, phenobarbital, and lamotrigine, with fever, rash, and eosinophilia. This may contribute to the morbidity of transplantation (Asconapé, 2002; Chabolla & Wszolek, 2006).

4. Azathioprine, mycophenolate mofetil, and muromonab (OKT3) metabolism is not significantly affected by AEDs (Chabolla & Wszolek, 2006).

5. Most transplant patients who experience one or two seizures during the peritransplantation period typically do not have long-term risk for recurrent seizures. A 1- to 3-month course of AED therapy is often sufficient to provide protection during a vulnerable period. Patients with potentially epileptogenic brain lesions or who are critically ill may need a longer course of AED therapy (Chabolla & Wszolek, 2006).

6. Most chemotherapeutic agents and immunosuppressant drugs have potential for bone marrow suppression. This side effect should be considered at the time of AED selection for epilepsy patients.

Antiepileptic Drugs in Patients on Chemotherapy or Immunosuppressive Therapy (Perucca, 2005; Drug Facts and Comparisons, 2007; van Breemen et al., 2007; Drugs' websites)

Acetazolamide

Acetazolamide is known to inhibit CYP3A4 and may decrease metabolism of other drugs and increase their plasma concentrations (Spina et al., 1996). This may amplify the toxicity of chemotherapeutic and immunosuppressive agents.

Carbamazepine

This drug is suboptimal in patients who receive chemotherapy or immunosuppressive therapy. Carbamazepine induces hepatic microsomal enzymes, which, in turn, accelerates the metabolism of other drugs, including many of the antineoplastic drugs. This drug is 76% protein bound in adults. Carbamazepine may interact with chemotherapeutic agents via different mechanisms. For example, myelosuppressive antineoplastic agents and radiation therapy possess hematologic toxicities similar to carbamazepine and should be used concomitantly with caution. Cisplatin and doxorubicin may increase the rate of carbamazepine metabolism because these antineoplastics induce hepatic microsomal enzymes (e.g., CYP3A). Dosage adjustments (either in carbamazepine or in antineoplastic agents) may be necessary, and closer monitoring of clinical and/or adverse effects is warranted when carbamazepine is used with any of the agents mentioned.

Eslicarbazepine Acetate

This is a less-than-ideal choice for patients receiving chemotherapy or immunosuppressive therapy due to hepatic metabolism and potential for drug interactions. Eslicarbazepine acetate can inhibit CYP2C19, which can cause increased plasma concentrations of drugs that are metabolized by this isoenzyme. In vivo studies suggest that eslicarbazepine acetate can induce CYP3A4, decreasing plasma concentrations of drugs that are metabolized by this isoenzyme.

Ethosuximide

This drug is a good choice for patients who require chemotherapy or immunosuppressive therapy.

Ezogabine

This drug is an acceptable choice for patients who require chemotherapy or immunosuppressive therapy with regard to drug interactions. However, it should be used only in the treatment of severe epilepsy refractory to other AEDs because of the risk of significant adverse effects.

Gabapentin

This drug is a good choice for patients with normal renal function who require chemotherapy or immunosuppressive therapy.

Lacosamide

This drug is a good choice for patients who require chemotherapy or immunosuppressive therapy.

Lamotrigine

Protein binding is 55% at plasma lamotrigine concentrations up to 10 µg/mL. It does not displace other AEDs from protein-binding sites. This is a less-than-ideal choice for patients receiving chemotherapy or immunosuppressive therapy due to hepatic metabolism and potential for drug interactions. Lamotrigine inhibits dihydrofolate reductase. Caution should be exercised when administering other drugs (e.g., fluorouracil or methotrexate), which may inhibit this enzyme.

Levetiracetam

This drug is a good choice for patients with normal renal function who receive chemotherapy or immunosuppressive therapy.

Oxcarbazepine

Oxcarbazepine and its metabolite 10-monohydroxy metabolite (MHD) produce a dose-related inhibition of CYP2C19 and induction of CYP3A4. The effectiveness of immunosuppressive medications such as cyclosporine, sirolimus, and tacrolimus could be decreased by the coadministration of oxcarbazepine (Rosche et al., 2001). This drug is suboptimal in patients who receive chemotherapy or immunosuppressive therapy for these reasons.

Perampanel

This drug is a reasonable choice for patients who receive chemotherapy or immunosuppressive therapy, although protein binding could be an issue. Perampanel is approximately 95% bound to plasma proteins.

Phenobarbital

This drug is suboptimal in patients who receive chemotherapy or immunosuppressive therapy. Phenobarbital accelerates the clearance of other drugs metabolized via hepatic microsomal enzymes (e.g., UGT enzymes, CYP2C-family enzymes, CYP3A-family enzymes, and CYP1A2). This drug is about 20%–45% bound to plasma proteins.

Phenytoin

This drug is suboptimal in patients who receive chemotherapy or immunosuppressive therapy. Mechanisms of drug interactions with phenytoin may be complex. In general, phenytoin is an inducer of the hepatic cytochrome P-450 microsomal enzymes including CYP3A4, CYP2C9, and CYP2C19 isoenzymes. This drug is about 90%–95% bound to plasma proteins.

Pregabalin

This drug is a reasonable choice in patients who receive chemotherapy or immunosuppressive therapy.

Rufinamide

This drug is an acceptable choice for patients who require chemotherapy or immunosuppressive therapy. Rufinamide is a weak inducer of the CYP 3A4 enzyme and can decrease exposure of drugs that are substrates of CYP 3A4. Only a small fraction of rufinamide (34%) is bound to serum proteins.

Tiagabine

Tiagabine does not inhibit or induce the hepatic CYP-450 microsomal enzymes or UGT. Tiagabine is extensively bound to plasma proteins (96%), mainly to serum albumin and α_1-acid glycoprotein.

Topiramate

Topiramate is not metabolized to a great extent. Protein binding range is 13%–41% to human plasma proteins. Topiramate may induce hepatic enzymes with dosages above 200 mg/day. Because of potential for interactions, high doses of this drug are less than ideal in patients who receive chemotherapy or immunosuppressive therapy.

Valproic Acid

This drug is suboptimal in patients who receive chemotherapy or immuno-suppressive therapy, because of interactions and enzyme inhibition. Valproic acid inhibits the activity of CYP2C9 and UGT at clinically relevant concentrations in human liver microsomes. Inhibition of CYP2C9 can explain some of the effects of valproic acid on the pharmacokinetics of other drugs. Valproic acid is about 90% protein bound.

Vigabatrin

This drug is an acceptable choice for patients who require chemotherapy or immunosuppressive therapy with regard to drug interactions. However, it should be used only in the treatment of severe epilepsy refractory to other AEDs because of the risk of visual field defect.

Zonisamide

This drug is a reasonable choice for patients who receive chemotherapy or immunosuppressive therapy, although protein binding could be an issue. In vitro data suggest that zonisamide does not inhibit or induce cytochrome P-450 enzymes or UGT. Zonisamide is not likely to interfere with the hepatic metabolic clearance of drugs metabolized by these enzyme systems. Zonisamide is approximately 40%–60% bound to human plasma proteins.

Recommended Antiepileptic Drugs in Epilepsy Patients on Chemotherapy or Immunosuppressive Therapy

1. **Generalized epilepsies:** Ethosuximide, levetiracetam, topiramate (low doses)
2. **Focal epilepsies:** Gabapentin, lacosamide, levetiracetam, topiramate (low doses)

References

Asconapé JJ. Some common issues in the use of antiepileptic drugs. *Seminars in Neurology*. 2002;22: 27–39.

Chabolla DR, Wszolek ZK. Pharmacologic management of seizures in organ transplant. *Neurology*. 2006;67: S34–S38.

Dasgupta A. Usefulness of monitoring free (unbound) concentrations of therapeutic drugs in patient management. *Clinica Chimica Acta*. 2007;377: 1–13.

Drug Facts and Comparisons. St. Louis: Wolters Kluwer Health/Facts & Comparisons, 2007.

Oberndorfer S, Piribauer M, Marosi C, Lahrmann H, Hitzenberger P, Grisold W. P-450 enzyme inducing and non-enzyme inducing antiepileptics in glioblastoma patients treated with standard chemotherapy. *Journal of Neuro-oncology*. 2005;72: 255–260.

Patsalos PN, Froscher W, Pisani F, van Rijn CM. The importance of drug interactions in epilepsy therapy. *Epilepsia*. 2002;43: 365–385.

Perucca E. Clinically relevant drug interactions with antiepileptic drugs. *British Journal of Clinical Pharmacology*. 2005;61: 246–255.

Perucca E. Optimizing antiepileptic drug treatment in tumoral epilepsy. *Epilepsia*. 2013;54 Suppl 9: 97–104.

Rosche J, Froscher W, Abendorth D, Liebel J. Possible oxcarbazepine interaction with cyclosporine serum levels: a single case study. *Clinical Neuropharmacology*. 2001;24: 113–116.

Spina E, Pisani F, Perucca E. Clinically significant pharmacokinetic drug interactions with carbamazepine. *Clinical Pharmacokinetics*. 1996;31: 198–214.

van Breemen MSM, Wilms EB, Vecht CJ. Epilepsy in patients with brain tumors: epidemiology, mechanisms, and management. *Lancet Neurology*. 2007;6: 421–430.

Vecht CJ, van Breemen M. Optimizing therapy of seizures in patients with brain tumors. *Neurology*. 2006;67: S10–S13.

Weller M, Stupp R, Wick W. Epilepsy meets cancer: when, why, and what to do about it? *Lancet Oncol* 2012;13(9): e375–e382.

Yap KY, Chui WK, Chan A. Drug interactions between chemotherapeutic regimens and antiepileptics. *Clin Ther* 2008;30(8): 1385–1407.

Sunovion. http://www.aptiom.com/2014

Eisai. http://www.banzel.com/2014

GSK. http://www.potiga.com/2014

UCB. http://www.vimpat.com/2014

Eisai. http://www.fycompa.com/2014

Lundbeck. http://www.sabril.net/2014

Chapter 20

Antiepileptic Drugs in Patients With Brain Tumors

Prophylactic anticonvulsant treatment is not advisable in brain tumor patients who have not experienced seizures. However, 30% to 50% of patients with brain tumors present with a seizure as their initial clinical manifestation, and up to 30% more will later develop seizures. Management of seizures associated with brain tumors requires consideration of several aspects, including a relatively high rate of recurrence after a first seizure, and more importantly, the possibility of adverse interactions between antiepileptic drugs (AEDs) and anticancer agents (see Chapter 19) and the disease itself. Most of the available data on selecting AEDs in patients with epilepsy and brain tumors originate from uncontrolled studies, and no large-scale well-designed randomized trial has been performed in this population. Therefore, a fully evidence-based approach to AED selection in patients with epilepsy secondary to brain tumors is not possible at the present time. Factors to be considered in making treatment selection include tolerability profile, comorbidities, drug-interaction potential, and cost. In other words, drug choice relies on both the theoretical advantages of pharmacokinetic properties and clinical judgment (Sperling & Ko, 2006; Perucca 2013).

There is no evidence that the efficacy ranking of currently available AEDs differs for patients with brain tumors compared with patients with focal seizures from other etiologies. However, limited evidence suggests that patients with brain tumors show increased susceptibility to the adverse effects of AEDs. This could be related to the underlying cerebral pathology, or to an interaction with anticancer therapy. The risk of AED-induced skin rashes, including Stevens-Johnson syndrome, is also increased in patients with brain tumors. The risk of interactions between AEDs and anticancer agents is a major concern (see Chapter 19). Although, some anticancer drugs commonly used in primary brain tumors (such as temozolomide) do not seem to be susceptible to enzyme induction, for others, such as irinotecan, etoposide, and tyrosine kinase inhibitors (e.g., erlotinib and imatinib), the increase in clearance caused by enzyme-inducer AEDs (e.g., carbamazepine, phenobarbital, phenytoin, and primidone) can be considerable and may need to be compensated by a corresponding increase in the dose of the anticancer agent (Perucca 2013). Valproic acid may favorably influence prognosis in patients with glioblastoma. Valproic acid has been found to induce apoptosis, autophagy, growth arrest, and cell differentiation of tumor cells, and also to inhibit tumor angiogenesis through inhibition of histone deacetylase and other mechanisms. These actions could contribute to inhibit tumor growth and might explain the apparent prolongation of survival in brain tumor patients (particularly, glioblastoma) treated with valproic acid. On the other hand, valproic acid also has intrinsic hematologic toxicity, particularly on platelet function, and inhibits a number of drug-metabolizing enzymes, causing an increase in the serum levels of some anticancer agents. Increased hematologic toxicity has been reported when valproic acid was given in combination with temozolomide and with other chemotherapeutic agents, including nitrosoureas, cisplatin, and etoposide. Valproic acid may cause thrombocytopenia, platelet dysfunction, and coagulation abnormalities, which represent a concern for patients in whom surgery is envisaged (see Chapter 18) (Perucca 2013). Levetiracetam, another potentially useful AED, has low interaction potential and good tolerability; it can be uptitrated relatively rapidly and also has parenteral formulation. In laboratory experiments, levetiracetam has been shown to enhance p53-mediated inhibition of MGMT, a DNA repair protein that has an important role in tumor cell resistance to alkylating agents and to sensitize glioblastoma cells to temozolomide; the clinical relevance of these findings is unknown. Oxcarbazepine and eslicarbazepine acetate have a relatively low interaction potential, but they do retain some enzyme-inducing and enzyme-inhibiting properties and may reduce the serum levels of certain anticancer drugs. Lamotrigine, perampanel, topiramate, and zonisamide need slow-dose titration, and they lack a parenteral formulation that could be a disadvantage in patients with brain tumor (Perucca 2013). Lacosamide has a parenteral formulation and is a good choice for patients who require chemotherapy with regard to drug interactions.

Recommended Antiepileptic Drugs in Epilepsy Patients with Brain Tumors

1. **Generalized epilepsies:** Valproate, levetiracetam
2. **Focal epilepsies:** Valproate, levetiracetam, lacosamide

Antiepileptic Drugs and Cancer

There is considerable debate about the relationship between AEDs and cancer, in particular, whether antiepileptic drugs promote or protect against cancer (Singh et al., 2005). Phenytoin and phenobarbital may induce carcinogenicity in rodent models. Phenobarbital promotes liver tumors in rats. Some early human epidemiological studies found an association between phenobarbital and hepatocellular carcinoma, and some subsequent studies suggested an association with lung cancer and brain tumor. Phenytoin causes lymphoid cell and liver tumors in rats. It has been associated with lymphoma, myeloma, and neuroblastoma in some human epidemiological studies (Murray et al., 1996). Carbamazepine results in a dose-related increase in the incidence of hepatocellular tumors in female rats and benign interstitial cell adenoma of testes in male rats. However, evidence for human carcinogenicity is inconsistent.

Valproate, in contrast, has been found to exert an antiproliferative effect on certain cancer cell lines both in vitro and in vivo (due to histone deacetylase inhibition). There are some reports of the use of valproate in human hematological and solid tumors (Olsen et al., 2004; Kaiser et al., 2006, Perucca, 2013).

Most new AEDs are probably safe with regard to carcinogenesis. There was no evidence of lacosamide related carcinogenicity in mice or rats. Vigabatrin showed no carcinogenic potential in mice or rats. There was no evidence of perampanel-related carcinogenicity in mice or rats. It is unknown whether gabapentin causes tumors in humans. A statistically significant increase in the incidence of pancreatic acinar cell adenomas and carcinomas has been found in male rats. However, in vitro testing has not shown mutagenic or clastogenic·changes. In carcinogenicity studies of pregabalin in mice, an unexpectedly high incidence of hemangiosarcoma was identified. Clinical experience during pregabalin premarketing development provides no direct means to assess its potential for inducing tumors in humans. An increase in the incidence of hepatocellular adenomas and carcinomas was observed in mice with eslicarbazepine acetate. In a one-year neonatal mouse study of ezogabine, a dose-related increase in the frequency of lung neoplasms (bronchio-alveolar carcinoma and/or adenoma) was observed. Increased incidences of tumors (benign bone tumors and/or hepatocellular adenomas and carcinomas) were observed in mice with rufinamide. Increased incidences of thyroid follicular adenomas were observed in rats with rufinamide. The incidence of hepatocellular adenoma in female rats and Leydig cell tumors in male rats was increased in a 2-year study with tiagabine. Finally, an increase in urinary bladder tumors was observed in mice given topiramate. The clinical significance of these findings in humans is unknown as mutagenesis is usually species specific (Singh et al., 2005; *Drug Facts and Comparisons*, 2007; Drugs' websites).

References

Drug Facts and Comparisons. St. Louis: Wolters Kluwer Health/Facts & Comparisons, 2007.

Kaiser M, Zavrski I, Sterz J, et al. The effects of the histone deacetylase inhibitor valproic acid on cell cycle, growth suppression and apoptosis in multiple myeloma. *Haematology*. 2006;91: 248–251.

Murray JC, Hill RM, Hegemier S, Hurwitz RL. Lymphoblastic lymphoma following prenatal exposure to phenytoin. *Journal of Pediatric Hematology and Oncology*. 1996;18(2): 241–243.

Olsen CM, Meussen-Elholm ET, Roste LS, Tauboll E. Antiepileptic drugs inhibit cell growth in the human breast cancer cell line MCF7. *Molecular and Cellular Endocrinology*. 2004;213: 173–179.

Perucca E. Optimizing antiepileptic drug treatment in tumoral epilepsy. *Epilepsia* 2013; 54 Suppl 9: 97–104.

Singh G, Driever PH, Sander JW. Cancer risk in people with epilepsy: the role of antiepileptic drugs. *Brain*. 2005;128: 7–17.

Sperling MR, Ko J. Seizures and brain tumors. *Seminars in Oncology*. 2006;33: 333–341.

Sunovion. http://www.aptiom.com/2014

Eisai. http://www.banzel.com/2014

GSK. http://www.potiga.com/2014

UCB. http://www.vimpat.com/2014

Eisai. http://www.fycompa.com/2014

Lundbeck. http://www.sabril.net/2014

Chapter 21

Antiepileptic Drugs in Patients With Stroke

Stroke and cerebrovascular lesions are the main cause of epilepsy in the elderly. The risk for development of epilepsy is 17-fold higher after stroke than in the age-matched general population; it is estimated that 10%–15% of stroke patients develop epilepsy (Ferro & Pinto, 2004). Seizures can be a presenting feature of acute stroke or may be a late complication.

Many similarities exist between cerebral ischemia and epilepsy regarding brain damage and autoprotective mechanisms that are activated following the injurious insult. Therefore, drugs that are effective in minimizing seizure-induced brain damage may also be useful in minimizing ischemic injury. On the other hand, some AEDs may have detrimental effects in stoke patients, and there is evidence that recovery is worse in patients treated with particular AEDs after stroke (Goldstein, 2000; Stepien et al., 2005).

There is no clinical evidence that prophylactic anticonvulsant treatment after stroke protects against the development of epilepsy. Transient AED therapy may be needed after a seizure occurring in the setting of an acute stroke (seizure occurring within the first week after a stroke), but prolonged, usually lifelong therapy is required after delayed seizures (seizure occurring more than 1 week after a stroke) due to high probability of seizure recurrence. When selecting an AED for a patient with stroke, one should consider the impact of an AED on comorbidity and comedications, the adverse effects, and cost among other factors (Stepien et al., 2005; Ryvlin & Montavont, 2006; Gilad 2012).

On the other hand, concern has been raised recently that some AEDs might increase the levels of serologic markers associated with an increased risk of vascular diseases (see Chapter 15 and Chapter 17). The duration of exposure to some AEDs may also predict acceleration of atherosclerosis. Based on these mechanisms, patients exposed to some AEDs could have an increased risk of vascular diseases such as stroke. In a recent study, the authors found that exposure to phenytoin was associated with a higher stroke risk as compared to carbamazepine. In addition, a longer duration and higher dosage of phenytoin demonstrated a dose–response relationship to increased stroke risk. Besides, studies have found that patients with epilepsy have higher stroke-related morbidity and mortality, which is probably related to AEDs, at least in part (Hsieh et al., 2013).

Benzodiazepines

Benzodiazepines may have potential detrimental effects in stroke patients (Schallert et al., 1986; Goldstein, 2000). In addition, adverse effects are significant in the elderly (Levy et al., 2002; *Drug Facts and Comparisons*, 2007). These are not recommended.

Carbamazepine

Carbamazepine has had some degree of neuroprotective activity in an ischemic/hypoxic model of neuronal injury (Willmore, 2005). However, due to enzyme induction and drug interactions, other AEDs may be a better choice (Levy et al., 2002; Parrish et al., 2006; *Drug Facts and Comparisons*, 2007). Because it induces cytochrome P-450 enzymes, doses of warfarin and other drugs (e.g., statins) will need to be increased.

Eslicarbazepine

Occurrence of hyponatremia is a potential problem. Besides, in vivo studies suggest that eslicarbazepine acetate can induce CYP3A4, decreasing plasma concentrations of drugs that are metabolized by this isoenzyme (e.g., simvastatin). Although the pharmacokinetics of eslicarbazepine are not affected by age independently, dose selection should take in consideration the greater frequency of renal impairment and medical comorbidities and drug therapies in the elderly patient.

Gabapentin

This drug does not demonstrate significant interaction with anticoagulants, antiplatelet agents, or other medications commonly prescribed in stroke patients, and its safety profile is relatively favorable (Stepien et al., 2005). Low target dosages (900–1200 mg/day) and slow titration over several weeks are appropriate in stroke patients (Stepien et al., 2005).

Lacosamide

This drug does not demonstrate significant interaction with anticoagulants, antiplatelet agents, or other medications commonly prescribed in stroke patients, and its safety profile is relatively favorable, but cardiovascular adverse effects and possibility of syncope should be kept in mind. The intravenous formulation can be used in patients with swallowing difficulty. Lacosamide treatment following status epilepticus attenuated neuronal cell loss and alterations in hippocampal neurogenesis in a rat electrical status epilepticus model (Licko et al., 2013).

Lamotrigine

This drug has fared well in randomized comparison trials in the elderly population (see Chapter 11) and is a good choice for stroke patients (Stepien et al., 2005). Lamotrigine also has had some degree of neuroprotective activity in an ischemic/hypoxic model of neuronal injury (Willmore, 2005). In addition, lamotrigine may help treat central poststroke pain (Vestergaard et al., 2001; Frese et al., 2006).

Levetiracetam

Due to its favorable pharmacokinetic profile and lack of drug interaction, this drug is a good choice for acute or chronic use. The intravenous formulation can be used in patients with swallowing difficulty. Levetiracetam may have some neuroprotective activity.

Oxcarbazepine

This drug is a reasonable choice, although the relatively common occurrence of hyponatremia is a potential problem. In dosages <900 mg daily, this drug does not demonstrate significant interaction with anticoagulants, antiplatelet agents, or other medications commonly prescribed in stroke patients, and its safety profile is relatively favorable (Stepien et al., 2005).

Perampanel

This drug does not demonstrate significant interaction with anticoagulants, antiplatelet agents, or other medications commonly prescribed in stroke patients, and its safety profile is relatively favorable. Elderly patients had an increased risk of falls compared to younger adults.

Phenobarbital

This is a suboptimal drug for chronic use and is mainly needed if status epilepticus occurs. Phenobarbital has had some degree of neuroprotective activity in an ischemic/hypoxic model of neuronal injury (Willmore, 2005). However, there are reports of delay in functional recovery in animal models of stroke or brain damage (Stepien et al., 2005). Phenobarbital may have potential detrimental effects in stoke patients (Goldstein, 2000). Importantly, due to adverse effects and drug interactions, use with precaution in elderly patients (Levy et al., 2002; *Drug Facts and Comparisons*, 2007).

Phenytoin

This drug is suboptimal for acute and long-term use, although the intravenous formulation offers acute treatment advantages. Hepatic enzyme induction, drug interactions, and its zero-order kinetics all pose difficulties (Levy et al., 2002; *Drug Facts and Comparisons*, 2007). Because it induces cytochrome P-450 enzymes, doses of warfarin and other drugs (e.g., statins) will need to be increased. Moreover, there are reports of alteration or delay in functional recovery in animal models of stroke or brain damage (Brailowsky et al., 1986; Stepien et al., 2005). Phenytoin may have detrimental effects in stroke patients as well (Goldstein, 2000). Likewise, prophylactic phenytoin may contribute to poor functional and cognitive outcomes in a dose-dependent manner after subarachnoid hemorrhage (Naidech et al., 2005). Phenytoin may also cause fever, which is associated with poor outcome and increased length of stay in direct proportion to the length of time the patient is febrile. However, phenytoin has demonstrated efficacy in treating central poststroke pain (Frese et al., 2006). Phenytoin has also shown neuroprotective activity in an ischemic/hypoxic model of neuronal injury (Willmore, 2005).

Pregabalin

There are little data regarding the use of this agent after stroke, but it has a good pharmacological profile.

Tiagabine

This drug is rarely used after stroke.

Topiramate

This drug is a reasonable choice, although drug interactions and cognitive side effects must be carefully monitored. Topiramate has neuroprotective properties and also reduces hemorrhagic incidence in focal cerebral ischemia in animal models; the human benefit has not been shown (Ferro & Pinto, 2004; Willmore, 2005).

Valproate

This agent has significant drug interactions, inhibits cytochrome P-450 enzymes, and binds extensively to plasma proteins. For these reasons, it is not an especially good choice for poststroke seizures. Acutely, it can be given intravenously if swallowing is not possible, which is an advantage. It may stabilize mood as well, which is an added benefit.

Zonisamide

This drug has a favorable pharmacological profile and is a reasonable choice. Zonisamide is an anticonvulsant compound that reduced infarct volume in ischemia-induced neuronal damage. Neuroprotective efficacy of zonisamide pretreatment was also shown in hypoxic/ischemic damage in neonatal rats (Ferro & Pinto, 2004; Willmore, 2005). Adverse effects are sometimes important, and the potential for renal stones should be remembered.

Recommended Antiepileptic Drugs in Epilepsy Patients With Stroke

Lacosamide, lamotrigine, levetiracetam, gabapentin

References

Brailowsky S, Knight RT, Efron R. Phenytoin increases the severity of cortical hemi-plegia in rats. *Brain Research*. 1986;376: 71–77.

Drug Facts and Comparisons. St. Louis: Wolters Kluwer Health/Facts & Comparisons, 2007.

Ferro JM, Pinto F. Poststroke epilepsy: epidemiology, pathophysiology and management. *Drugs and Aging*. 2004;21: 639–653.

Frese A, Husstedt IW, Ringelstein EB, Evers S. Pharmacologic treatment of central post-stroke pain. *Clinical Journal of Pain*. 2006;22: 252–260.

Gilad R. Management of seizures following a stroke: what are the options? *Drugs Aging*. 2012; 29(7): 533–538.

Goldstein LB. Rehabilitation and recovery after stroke. *Current Treatment Options in Neurology*. 2000;2: 319–328.

Hsieh CY, Lai EC, Yang YH, Lin SJ. Comparative stroke risk of antiepileptic drugs in patients with epilepsy. *Epilepsia*. 2013;54(1): 172–180.

Levy RH, Mattson RH, Meldrum BS, Perucca E. *Antiepileptic Drugs*. 5th ed. Philadelphia: Lippincott Williams & Wilkins, 2002.

Licko T, Seeger N, Zellinger C, Russmann V, Matagne A, Potschka H. Lacosamide treatment following status epilepticus attenuates neuronal cell loss and alterations in hippocampal neurogenesis in a rat electrical status epilepticus model. *Epilepsia*. 2013; 54(7): 1176–1185.

Naidech AM, Kreiter KT, Janjua N, et al. Phenytoin exposure is associated with functional and cognitive disability after subarachnoid hemorrhage. *Stroke*. 2005;36: 583–587.

Parrish RH, Pazdur DE, O'Donnell PJ. Effect of carbamazepine initiation and discontinuation on antithrombotic control in a patient receiving warfarin: case report and review of the literature. *Pharmacotherapy*. 2006;26: 1650–1653.

Ryvlin P, Montavont A, Nighoghossian N. Optimizing therapy of seizures in stroke patients. *Neurology*. 2006;67: S3–S9.

Schallert T, Hernandez TD, Barth TM. Recovery of function after brain damage: severe and chronic disruption by diazepam. *Brain Research*. 1986;379: 104–111.

Stepien K, Tomaszewski M, Czuczwar SJ. Profile of anticonvulsant activity and neuroprotective effects of novel and potential antiepileptic drugs—an update. *Pharmacology Reports*. 2005;57: 719–733.

Vestergaard K, Andersen G, Gottrup H, et al. Lamotrigine for central poststroke pain: a randomized controlled trial. *Neurology*. 2001;23;56: 184–190.

Willmore LJ. Antiepileptic drugs and neuroprotection: current status and future roles. *Epilepsy and Behavior*. 2005;7(Suppl 3): S25–S28.

Chapter 22

Antiepileptic Drugs in Patients With Preexisting Psychiatric Problems or Learning Disabilities

Although most people with epilepsy lead normal lives, neurobehavioral problems are found in a large proportion of patients. Higher rates of psychopathology are observed in people with epilepsy relative to the general population, to other neurological control groups, and to people with chronic non-neurological disorders. This largely reflects the effect of uncontrolled epilepsy and the underlying brain injury, which predispose patients to depression, anxiety, and other psychiatric symptoms. In particular, increased psychopathology is common in patients with refractory temporal lobe epilepsy (TLE). Depression is the most frequent type of psychiatric disorder identified in patients with epilepsy, with prevalence of up to 50% in some studies (Mendez et al., 1986). Epidemiological studies have identified a variety of psychoses in up to 9% of epilepsy patients. Likewise, patients with epilepsy commonly report anxiety and, finally, the risk of suicide in patients with epilepsy is estimated to be 4 to 5 times greater than that of the general population, and a higher risk is found in TLE (Kanner & Palac, 2002). The causes of psychopathology in epilepsy are multifactorial and include genetic predisposition, biological risk factors, iatrogenic causes (e.g., antiepileptic drugs), and other causes. A bidirectional relationship between psychosis or depression and epilepsy has been suggested in the literature. For example, similar neurotransmitter alterations may underlie both depression and epilepsy (Yan et al., 1998). Although the clinical manifestations of psychiatric disorders in epilepsy are often indistinguishable from those of nonepileptic patients, certain types of depression and psychotic disorders may present with clinical characteristics that are particular to those of patients with epilepsy. These include postictal psychosis, alternate psychosis (or forced normalization), and certain forms of interictal depressive disorders.

Some antiepileptic drugs (AEDs) are also psychotropic agents with positive or negative effects. The psychotropic effects of AEDs in people with epilepsy are, however, variable and unpredictable. Unfortunately, a history of psychiatric illness may be a risk factor for a negative psychotropic effect by an AED. Thus, the beneficial psychotropic effects seen with AEDs in the general nonepileptic population may be less apparent in epilepsy patients. However, for example, it would be reasonable to prescribe an appropriate AED with

Box 22.1	Approved Psychiatric Indications for Antiepileptic Drugs
Benzodiazepines	Anxiety disorders, alcohol withdrawal, insomnia
Carbamazepine	Bipolar disorder, mania
Valproate	Bipolar disorder, mania and bipolar disorder, mixed
Lamotrigine	Bipolar disorder, maintenance
Pregabalin	Generalized anxiety disorder

Adapted from: Kaufman KR. Antiepileptic drugs in the treatment of psychiatric disorders. *Epilepsy Behav* 2011; 21(1): 1–11.

anxiolytic potential in a patient with preexisting anxiety disorder. For instance, pregabalin, and to a lesser extent gabapentin, are effective in anxiety disorders and pregabalin is in fact licensed for the treatment of generalized anxiety disorder (Box 22.1). On the other hand, the treating physician should be aware of the possibility of aggravating anxiety symptomatology when prescribing certain AEDs to patients with epilepsy (Box 22.2). Besides, use of sedating doses and combinations of AEDs that can impair cognitive and behavioral functions should be avoided in all patients (Nadkarni & Devinsky,

Box 22.2 Psychiatric Adverse Effects of Antiepileptic Drugs in Patients With Preexisting Psychopathologies

Preexisting Psychopathology	Precautions in Using Antiepileptic Drugs	Possible Adverse Effects
Dysthymia	Phenobarbital, tiagabine, levetiracetam, topiramate, vigabatrin, zonisamide	Major depression
Paranoia	Phenytoin, ethosuximide, topiramate, vigabatrin, zonisamide	Schizophrenic psychosis
Dysphoria	Levetiracetam, zonisamide	Aggression
Agitation	Lamotrigine	Insomnia, anxiety, hypomania
Anxiety	Levetiracetam, zonisamide	Agitation or aggression
Attention-deficit hyperactivity disorder	Phenobarbital, primidone, valproate, gabapentin, topiramate, lamotrigine, levetiracetam	Deterioration of attention and behavior
Hyperactivity	Benzodiazepines, phenobarbital (usually in children or elderly)	Paradoxical central nervous system stimulation
Learning disability	Phenobarbital, topiramate, zonisamide	Behavioral disorders, impaired cognition
Developmental disabilities with cognitive dysfunction	Phenobarbital, topiramate, benzodiazepines, gabapentin, zonisamide	Worsening of intellectual disabilities

From Tiffin and Perini (2001), Devinsky (2004), Schubert (2005), Schmitz (2006), Aldendamp et al. (2006), Brodtkorb and Mula (2006), and Smith (2006).

2005; Schmitz, 2006; Kaufman, 2011; Bialer, 2012; Kimiskidis & Valeta, 2012). When prescribing an AED for a patient with epilepsy, preexisting psychiatric problems or learning disabilities, drug-drug interactions and adverse effects of the AED should be considered (Boxes 22.2, 22.3, and 22.4). The treating physician should consider which AED might best help the patient in maximizing seizure control and minimizing psychiatric symptoms.

Last, all AEDs have the potential to cause adverse psychiatric effects. Antiepileptic drugs increase the risk of suicidal thoughts or behavior in patients taking these drugs for any indication. The increased risk of suicidal thoughts or behavior with AEDs is observed as early as 1 week after starting treatment with AEDs and persists for the duration of treatment. Patients treated with *any AED for any indication* should be monitored for the emergence or worsening of depression, suicidal thoughts or behavior, and/or any unusual changes in mood or behavior. However, in the authors' experience, some agents are more apt to do so than others. We have observed the greatest incidence of psychiatric side effects with phenobarbital, primidone, levetiracetam, topiramate, and zonisamide. Patients and their families should be cautioned about potential psychiatric adverse effects when these agents are used, so that problems can be promptly addressed should they occur. (Box 22.3 and Box 22.4)

Note: Sexual dysfunction due to AEDs is common and may have psychiatric consequences:

1. Enzyme-inducing AEDs, such as carbamazepine, phenytoin, phenobarbital, primidone, and oxcarbazepine and topiramate in high doses, can increase sex hormone–binding globulin, reduce free (bioactive)

Box 22.3 Recommended Antiepileptic Drugs in Epilepsy Patients With Preexisting Psychiatric, Learning, and Behavioral Problems

Preexisting Psychopathology	Recommended Antiepileptic Drugs
Depression	Valproate, carbamazepine, lamotrigine, gabapentin, pregabalin
Mania	Valproate, carbamazepine, oxcarbazepine, lamotrigine
Bipolar disorder	Valproate, carbamazepine, lamotrigine, oxcarbazepine
Aggression and agitation	Valproate, carbamazepine, phenytoin
Anxiety disorders	Pregabalin, gabapentin (social anxiety disorder)
Binge-eating disorder	Topiramate, zonisamide
Learning disability	Carbamazepine, lamotrigine, levetiracetam
Attention-deficit-hyperactivity disorder	Levetiracetam, lamotrigine, carbamazepine, oxcarbazepine, gabapentin

From Nadkarni and Devinsky (2005), Brodtkorb and Mula (2006), Schubert (2005), Schmitz (2006), Mula et al. (2007), Tassone et al. (2007), Kaufman (2011), Bialer (2012), and Kimiskidis and Valeta (2012).

Box 22.4 Psychiatric Averse Effects of Antiepileptic Drugs

Antiepileptic Drug	Psychiatric Adverse Effects	Note
Acetazolamide	Irritability, libido decrease	—
Benzodiazepines	Depression, paradoxical central nervous system stimulation (hostility, nightmares, talkativeness, excitement, mania, tremors, sleep disturbances, increased muscle spasticity, acute rage reactions, anxiety, restlessness, euphoria, and hyperreflexia, particularly in psychiatric patients and hyperactive children), dependence, sexual dysfunction, and libido decrease	Most of the adverse effects are dose dependent. Tolerance may develop to these effects. Benzodiazepine therapy should be discontinued if any of the signs of paradoxical CNS excitement occur.
Carbamazepine	Irritability, agitation, depression, talkativeness, sexual dysfunction	—
Eslicarbazepine acetate	Depression, insomnia	—
Ethosuximide	Aggression, irritability, restlessness or hyperactivity, depression (with suicidal ideations), insomnia, euphoria, and rarely: nightmares, emotional lability, paranoia-type psychosis, libido increase	Rare adverse effects are more likely to occur in patients who have previously shown abnormal psychological reactions.
Ezogabine	Confusional state, psychotic symptoms, hallucinations, abnormal thinking, dependence	These effects are dose-related and generally appear within the first 8 weeks of treatment. Rapid titration at greater than the recommended doses appeared to increase the risk of psychosis and hallucinations.
Felbamate	Somnolence, insomnia, nervousness, aggression, anxiety, depression, abnormal thinking, hallucination, psychosis, emotional lability, euphoria, mania	Adverse psychiatric effects have caused discontinuance of the drug in about 2% of adults and 1% of children.
Gabapentin	Irritability, agitation, anxiety and hostility, hyperkinesia, abnormal thinking	All more common in children with disabilities. Pediatric patients should be monitored closely for central nervous system adverse effects.
Lacosamide	Depression, confusional state, aggression, agitation, hallucination, insomnia, psychotic disorder	—
Lamotrigine	Insomnia, irritability (usually in children with disabilities), depression, anxiety, emotional lability	—

(continued)

Box 22.4 (Continued)

Antiepileptic Drug	Psychiatric Adverse Effects	Note
Levetiracetam	Anxiety, depression, irritability, agitation, aggression, anger, insomnia, apathy, depersonalization, emotional lability, hyperkinesia, hallucinations, hostility, personality disorders, psychosis, psychotic depression	May be seen at any dose. Counsel patients and caregivers of the need to monitor for the emergence of anger, aggression, hostility, unusual changes in mood, personality, or behavior.
Oxcarbazepine	Emotional lability, insomnia, abnormal thinking	Usually occurs with dosages > 1200 mg/day
Perampanel	Hostility, aggression, irritability, anger, anxiety, paranoia, mood changes, confusional state	These effects are dose-related and generally appear within the first 6 weeks of treatment. Counsel patients and caregivers of the need to monitor for the emergence of anger, aggression, hostility, unusual changes in mood, personality, or behavior.
Phenobarbital	Aggression, depression, emotional lability, irritability, anxiety, sexual dysfunction and libido decrease, dependence, paradoxical CNS stimulation (adverse behavioral reactions, hyperactivity, nightmares, insomnia), or exacerbation of preexisting hyperactivity in some children	Geriatric patients have experienced agitation, excitation, or depression.
Phenytoin	Depression, sexual dysfunction including libido decrease, impotence	The severity of these adverse reactions increases as serum concentrations of phenytoin increase.
Pregabalin	Abnormal thinking, euphoria, impotence, libido decrease, insomnia, dependence	The majority of these adverse events are mild to moderate in intensity and dose dependent.
Rufinamide	Psychomotor hyperactivity, anxiety, aggression, behavioral disturbance, depression	—
Tiagabine	Depression, irritability, hostility, anxiety, abnormal thinking, insomnia	Slow initial titration may help to minimize these central nervous system effects.
Topiramate	Depression, psychomotor impairment, irritability, nervousness, anxiety, emotional lability, depersonalization, insomnia, hallucinations, euphoria, psychosis, impotence, libido decrease	Most psychiatric adverse effects usually occur with dosages > 200 mg/day.

(continued)

Box 22.4 (Continued)		
Antiepileptic Drug	**Psychiatric Adverse Effects**	**Note**
Valproate	Depression, agitation, nervousness, hallucinations, euphoria	Mental status changes (e.g., depression, agitation) are most likely to occur in children.
Vigabatrin	Insomnia, irritability, depression, confusional state, abnormal behaviour, abnormal thinking, abnormal dream	—
Zonisamide	Aggression, irritability, nervousness, anxiety, depression, insomnia, emotional lability, schizophrenic/ schizophreniform behaviour	Most psychiatric adverse effects usually occur with dosages > 300 mg/day.

All antiepileptic drugs may increase the risk of suicidal thoughts or behavior in patients taking these drugs for any indication.

From: Levy et al. (2002); *Drug Facts and Comparisons* (2007); Kaufman (2011); drugs' websites.

testosterone, and thereby reduce libido and impair sexual function (Harden, 2006).

2. Other AEDs, including acetazolamide, benzodiazepines, pregabalin, and topiramate, may cause sexual dysfunction as well.

3. Sexual dysfunction is not common with ethosuximide, gabapentin, lamotrigine, levetiracetam, tiagabine, valproate, and zonisamide (*Drug Facts and Comparisons,* 2007). However, study of sexual function with these drugs is limited.

References

Aldenkamp AP, Arzimanoglou A, Reijs R, Van Mil S. Optimizing therapy of seizures in children and adolescents with ADHD. *Neurology.* 2006;67: S49–S51.

Bialer M. Why are antiepileptic drugs used for nonepileptic conditions? *Epilepsia.* 2012;53 Suppl 7: 26–33.

Brodtkorb E, Mula M. Optimizing therapy of seizures in adult patients with psychiatric comorbidity. *Neurology.* 2006;67: S39–S44.

Devinsky O. Therapy for neurobehavioral disorders in epilepsy. *Epilepsia.* 2004;45(Suppl 2): 34–40.

Drug Facts and Comparisons. St. Louis: Wolters Kluwer Health/Facts & Comparisons, 2007.

Harden CL. Sexuality in men and women with epilepsy. *CNS Spectrums.* 2006; 11(8 Suppl 9): 13–18.

Kanner AM, Palac S. Neuropsychiatric complications of epilepsy. *Current Neurology and Neuroscience Reports.* 2002;2: 365–372.

Kaufman KR. Antiepileptic drugs in the treatment of psychiatric disorders. *Epilepsy Behav.* 2011; 21(1): 1–11.

Kimiskidis VK, ValetaT. Epilepsy and anxiety: epidemiology, classification, aetiology, and treatment. *Epileptic Disord*. 2012; 14(3): 248–256.

Levy RH, Mattson RH, Meldrum BS, Perucca E. *Antiepileptic Drugs*. 5th ed. Philadelphia: Lippincott Williams & Wilkins, 2002.

Mendez MF, Cummings JL, Benson DF. Depression in epilepsy: significance and phenomenology. *Archives of Neurology*. 1986;43: 766–770.

Mula M, Pini S, Cassano GB. The role of anticonvulsant drugs in anxiety disorders: a critical review of the evidence. *Journal of Clinical Psychopharmacology*. 2007;27: 263–272.

Nadkarni S, Devinsky O. Psychotropic effects of antiepileptic drugs. *Epilepsy Currents*. 2005;5(5): 176–181.

Schmitz B. Effects of antiepileptic drugs on mood and behavior. *Epilepsia*. 2006;47(Suppl 2): 28–33.

Schubert R. Attention deficit disorder and epilepsy. *Pediatric Neurology*. 2005;32: 1–10.

Smith MC. Optimizing therapy of seizures in children and adolescents with developmental disabilities. *Neurology*. 2006;67: S52–S55.

Tassone DM, Boyce E, Guyer J, Nuzum D. Pregabalin: a novel gamma aminobutiric acid analogue in the treatment of neuropathic pain, partial-onset seizures, and anxiety disorders. *Clinical Therapy*. 2007;29: 26–48.

Tiffin PA, Perini AF. The use of antiepileptic drugs in learning disabled people with epilepsy: an audit of adult in-patients in a treatment and continuing care service. *Seizure*. 2001;10: 500–504.

Yan QS, Dailey JW, Steenbergen JL, et al. Anticonvulsant effect of enhancement of noradrenergic transmission in the superior colliculus in genetically epilepsy-prone rats (GEPRs). A microinjection study. *Brain Research*. 1998;780: 199.

Sunovion. http://www.aptiom.com/2014

Eisai. http://www.banzel.com/2014

GSK. http://www.potiga.com/2014

UCB. http://www.vimpat.com/2014

Eisai. http://www.fycompa.com/2014

Lundbeck. http://www.sabril.net/2014

Chapter 23

Antiepileptic Drugs and Cognition

Cognition comprises a broad range of functions, such as attention, intelligence, visual memory, and language skills, among others. Problems with cognition can be manifested as reductions in attention, IQ, language and perceptual skills, executive functions including problem solving, verbal and visual memory, and motor speed. Treating a patient with epilepsy involves more than just treating seizures. Many patients have associated learning and cognitive problems that lead to significant difficulties at school or work. Educational underachievement is considered to be the greatest academic complication in a child with epilepsy. Children with epilepsy, even those with normal intelligence, often experience educational difficulties more often than unaffected children. These educational problems tend to persist into adulthood and are sometimes manifested as underemployment (Vinayan, 2006; Hermann et al., 2010).

The causes of cognitive impairment in patients with epilepsy include effect of ongoing seizures, underlying structural brain lesions, and adverse effects of AEDs. The effect of AEDs on the learning process and cognitive function in a patient with epilepsy is double-edged. AEDs can control epileptic seizures, leading to improvement in cognitive functions and other learning processes. On the other hand, AEDS can adversely affect learning processes and cognition. Although the cognitive effects of AEDs are generally modest, these effects at times have clinical significance (Brunbech & Sabers, 2002; Meador, 2006; Vinayan, 2006).

Therefore, two considerations are important when treating someone with epilepsy. Seizures must be prevented, but side effects, especially cognitive ones, should be avoided. This is especially important for children who are in a critical period of brain development, whose major "occupation" is learning. Maintaining cognitive abilities is important for everyone else because everyone requires good mental function; this is especially important for people whose vocations require high-level cognitive processing. All AEDs have the potential for detrimentally affecting cognitive function. These effects are especially common with higher doses of AEDs or with polytherapy. Besides, cognitive effects exerted by an AED could vary depending on factors linked to patient characteristics and individual susceptibility. Of the older AEDs, phenobarbital, primidone and benzodiazepines produce the greatest degree of learning and cognitive impairments. Phenobarbital may influence IQ and have deleterious effects on attention; it can reduce processing efficiency. Phenobarbital is considered to have worse cognitive effects than valproate or carbamazepine.

Phenytoin and high doses of valproate have also been reported to cause impairment in memory and learning processes. The cognitive effects associated with phenytoin may be more obvious but are generally restricted to visually guided motor functions. Valproate has been suggested to be preferable to carbamazepine, phenobarbital, and topiramate. However, attention dysfunction was more common with valproic acid than ethosuximide. Cognitive problems due to carbamazepine are not common, but high doses can impair functions. Carbamazepine has a cognitive profile that is worse than levetiracetam and lamotrigine but better than phenytoin. Oxcarbazepine and gabapentin have benign cognitive profiles. Lamotrigine and levetiracetam have been shown to have a favorable cognitive profile in comparison with other AEDs. Among newer AEDs, topiramate and zonisamide have the greatest potential to impair cognition, but with high doses, all can cause problems (Brunbech & Sabers, 2002; Meador, 2006; Vinayan, 2006; *Drug Facts and Comparisons*, 2007; Kothare & Kaleyias, 2007; Eddy et al., 2011).

It should be emphasized that cognition is only one consideration when choosing an AED. Efficacy, the patient's profile, other side effects and even cost must also be taken into account. Whenever possible, it is prudent to use the lowest effective dose of the AED, titrate upward slowly, and employ monotherapy. Keep in mind, however, that a patient's perception of cognitive adverse effects of therapy might be more related to mood than to actual cognitive performance. Patients who report having trouble with memory or learning might actually be depressed. If there is evidence of a mood disorder, its treatment should be considered. It is also important to reassess the frequency and severity of the seizures and the efficacy of the AEDs in use, as well as to assess the adverse effects of the disease in addition to the adverse effects of treatment at each visit (Hermann et al., 2010). (Box 23.1)

Box 23.1 Cognitive Adverse Effects of Antiepileptic Drugs

Antiepileptic Drug	Cognitive Adverse Effects	Note
Acetazolamide	Drowsiness, confusion	Uncommon
Benzodiazepines	Drowsiness, confusion, paradoxical central nervous system stimulation	Most of these side effects are dose dependent.
Carbamazepine	Drowsiness, confusion, impaired attention, impaired motor tasks	Seen mainly with high levels
Eslicarbazepine acetate	Memory impairment, disturbance in attention, amnesia, aphasia, speech disorder, slowness of thought, disorientation, and psychomotor retardation	These side effects are dose dependent.

(continued)

Box 23.1 (Continued)

Antiepileptic Drug	Cognitive Adverse Effects	Note
Ethosuximide	Drowsiness, confusion, and rarely impaired cognition	
Ezogabine	Memory impairment, disturbance in attention, aphasia, amnesia	
Felbamate	Drowsiness, confusion	Often makes patients more alert with improvement in cognition
Gabapentin	Amnesia, mental depression, drowsiness, impaired cognition	Minimal or some cognitive adverse effects. All are more common in children with disabilities.
Lacosamide	Memory impairment, disturbance in attention	Often, not severe.
Lamotrigine	Confusion, drowsiness	Minimal cognitive adverse effects except at high dosages above 400 to 500 mg/day.
Levetiracetam	Drowsiness, amnesia	Cognitive adverse effects are minimal with dosages of 1000 to 3000 mg/day.
Oxcarbazepine	Confusion, drowsiness, impaired concentration and cognition, speech problems	Most adverse effects occur with dosages above 1200 mg/day.
Perampanel	Memory impairment, dysarthria	
Phenobarbital	Impaired cognition, memory and attention, mental slowing, drowsiness, confusion, paradoxical CNS stimulation or exacerbation of preexisting hyperactivity in some children	Potentially significant cognitive adverse effects. Children treated chronically with phenobarbital may experience subtle cognitive decline. Geriatric patients have experienced agitation, excitation, depression, or confusion.
Phenytoin	Drowsiness, confusion, impaired attention, reduction in motor speed and problem solving	Some cognitive adverse effects. The severity of these adverse reactions increases as serum concentrations of phenytoin increase.

(continued)

Box 23.1 (Continued)

Antiepileptic Drug	Cognitive Adverse Effects	Note
Pregabalin	Difficulty with concentration/attention, drowsiness, confusion, amnesia	Some cognitive adverse effects. The majority of these adverse events are mild to moderate in intensity and dose dependent.
Rufinamide	Rare (not specified)	
Tiagabine	Impaired cognition, impaired concentration, drowsiness, confusion, amnesia	Minimal cognitive adverse effects. Slow initial titration may minimize these effects.
Topiramate	Psychomotor impairment, impaired cognition and language (word finding difficulty, memory impairment), drowsiness, confusion	Potentially significant cognitive adverse effects. Most adverse effects usually occur with dosages above 200 mg/day, but can be seen with low doses. Slow titration minimizes these effects.
Valproate	Drowsiness	Some cognitive adverse effects. Mental status changes are most likely to occur in children.
Vigabatrin	Memory impairment, disturbance in attention, expressive language disorder	
Zonisamide	Confusion, drowsiness, difficulty concentrating, impaired cognition (memory), mental slowing and psychomotor impairment, speech impairment (speech abnormalities and difficulty in verbal expression)	Some cognitive adverse effects. Most adverse effects usually occur with dosages above 300 mg/day.

From Mendez et al. (1986), Yan et al. (1998), Kanner and Palac (2002), Nadkarni and Devinsky (2005), Drugs' websites.

References

Brunbech L, Sabers A. Effect of antiepileptic drugs on cognitive function in individuals with epilepsy. *Drugs*. 2002;62: 593–604.

Drug Facts and Comparisons. St. Louis: Wolters Kluwer Health/Facts & Comparisons, 2007.

Eddy CM, Rickards HE, Cavanna AE, The cognitive impact of antiepileptic drugs. *Ther Adv Neurol Disord*. 2011;4(6): 385–407.

Hermann B, Meador KJ, Gaillard WD, Cramer JA. Cognition across the lifespan: antiepileptic drugs, epilepsy, or both? *Epilepsy Behav*. 2010;17(1): 1–5.

Kanner AM, Palac S. Neuropsychiatric complications of epilepsy. *Current Neurology and Neuroscience Reports*, 2002;2: 365–372.

Kothare SV, Kaleyias J. The adverse effects of antiepileptic drugs in children. *Expert Opinion on Drug Safety*. 2007;6: 251–265.

Meador KJ. Cognitive and behavioral effects of AEDs. *Epilepsy Research*. 2006;68: 63–67.

Mendez MF, Cummings JL, Benson DF. Depression in epilepsy: significance and phenomenology. *Archives of Neurology*. 1986;43: 766–770.

Nadkarni S, Devinsky O. Psychotropic effects of antiepileptic drugs. *Epilepsy Currents*, 2005;5(5): 176–181.

Vinayan KP. Epilepsy, antiepileptic drugs and educational problems. *Indian Pediatrics*, 2006;43: 786–794.

Yan QS, Dailey JW, Steenbergen JL, et al. Anticonvulsant effect of enhancement of noradrenergic transmission in the superior colliculus in genetically epilepsy-prone rats (GEPRs). A microinjection study. *Brain Research*, 1998;780: 199.

Sunovion. http://www.aptiom.com/2014

Eisai. http://www.banzel.com/2014

GSK. http://www.potiga.com/2014

UCB. http://www.vimpat.com/2014

Eisai. http://www.fycompa.com/2014

Lundbeck. http://www.sabril.net/2014

Chapter 24

Antiepileptic Drugs in Patients With Migraine Headaches

Two disorders are comorbid if they occur in the same person more frequently than by chance alone. Migraine and epilepsy appear to be comorbid. The prevalence of epilepsy in persons with migraine ranges from 1% to 17% with a median of 5.9%, substantially higher than the population prevalence of epilepsy (Andermann & Andermann, 1987). The reported frequency of migraine in epileptic populations ranges from 8.4% to 24.0% (Marks & Ehrenberg, 1993; Ottman & Lipton, 1996; Stevenson, 2006).

Migraine and epilepsy share several clinical features and may share some common pathophysiological mechanisms. Both are considered to be disorders of neuronal hyperexcitability. In addition, similar triggering factors have been identified for both migraine and epilepsy (e.g., menses, alcohol, and sleep deprivation). An imbalance between excitatory glutamate-mediated transmission and GABA-mediated inhibition in specific brain areas has been postulated in both conditions. Moreover, abnormal activation of voltage-operated ionic channels has been implicated in both migraine and epilepsy (Aurora et al., 1999; Koch et al., 2005; Calabresi et al., 2007).

Some antiepileptic drugs (AEDs) are effective in reducing migraine frequency. The AEDs that are most effective therapies for migraine prophylaxis in adults include valproate and topiramate. Indeed, these agents are prescribed as first-line agents for prophylactic treatment of migraine headaches, whether epilepsy is comorbid or not. Gabapentin is also somewhat effective and may be considered as a second-line therapy in migraine prophylaxis (Modi & Lowder, 2006; Calabresi et al., 2007; D'Amico, 2007). On the other hand, some AEDs have no demonstrable effect on migraine, and others may cause headaches as a side effect. Therefore, caution should be exercised before over-relating epilepsy and migraines; while some features are shared, the differences probably outweigh the similarities.

Gabapentin

Gabapentin has been evaluated in controlled trials and demonstrated conflicting results for migraine prophylaxis (Mathew et al., 2001; Buchanan & Ramadan, 2006; Modi & Lowder, 2006; Pierangeli et al., 2006; Calabresi et al., 2007; D'Amico, 2007; Linde et al., 2013).

Lamotrigine

The efficacy of lamotrigine in migraine prevention is uncertain. Open-label studies suggest that it may be efficacious in migraine with aura (Buchanan & Ramadan, 2006; D'Amico, 2007), but the only controlled double-blind study that has been performed did not show efficacy in migraine prophylaxis (Steiner et al., 1997). Further study is required.

Levetiracetam

In a small prospective, randomized, double-blind, parallel-group trial, leve-tiracetam 1000 mg/day was significantly superior to placebo in reducing headache frequency, as well as in the proportion of responders. The same trial examined levetiracetam 1000 mg/day versus topiramate 100 mg/day and found a small difference favoring topiramate in headache frequency (de Tommaso et al., 2007).

Pregabalin

Pregabalin is one of the gabapentinoids and has some efficacy and safety for migraine prophylaxis (Buchanan & Ramadan, 2006), but more research is desirable (Linde et al., 2013).

Topiramate

Topiramate is efficacious and safe in migraine prevention. It is considered as the best AED for migraine treatment by the authors and has been shown in double-blind placebo-controlled trials to be effective for migraine prevention (Buchanan & Ramadan, 2006; Modi & Lowder, 2006; Pierangeli et al., 2006; Calabresi et al., 2007; D'Amico, 2007; Diener et al., 2007). In one study, the responder rate among patients with migraine was significantly greater with topiramate at 50 mg/day (39%, $P = 0.01$), 100 mg/day (49%, $P < 0.001$), and 200 mg/day (47%, $P < 0.001$) versus placebo (23%). Reductions in number of migraine days were significant for the 100 mg/day (p = 0.003) and 200-mg/day (p < 0.001) topiramate groups (Brandes et al., 2004). A meta-analysis demonstrated that topiramate in a 100 mg/day dosage is effective in reducing headache frequency and reasonably well tolerated (Linde et al., 2013).

Valproate (Valproic Acid, Divalproex Sodium)

Valproate has been studied in migraine as well, and its efficacy has been established. In one study, the mean reductions in 4-week migraine headache rate were 1.2 headaches per 4 weeks (from a baseline mean of 4.4) in the extended-release divalproex sodium group and 0.6 headache per 4 weeks (from a baseline mean of 4.2) in the placebo group (p = 0.006); reductions with extended-release divalproex sodium were significantly greater than with placebo in all three 4-week segments of the treatment period (Freitag et al., 2002). This result is not striking but is significant. This drug is a good choice for patients with migraine and comorbid bipolar disease or epilepsy (Buchanan & Ramadan, 2006; Modi & Lowder, 2006; Pierangeli et al., 2006; Calabresi et al., 2007; D'Amico, 2007).

Zonisamide

Preliminary data suggest that it may be effective for this indication (Ashkenazi et al., 2006). One trial examined zonisamide (200 mg/day) versus topiramate (100 mg/day) and found no significant difference between them in reduction of headache frequency. Headache severity was reduced significantly better by zonisamide (Mohammadininejad et al., 2011).

It is noteworthy to mention that evidence suggests that there may be a role for AEDs, especially valproate, topiramate, and gabapentin, in the prevention of cluster headaches as well (D'Amico, 2007; Pascual et al., 2007).

Finally, it should be mentioned that chronic headache may occur in some patients treated with carbamazepine or oxcarbazepine (Palmieri, 2007). The cause is uncertain. In the authors' experience, this is occasionally dose related, but usually use of the drug must discontinue for the headache to disappear.

Recommended Antiepileptic Drugs in Epilepsy Patients With Migraine Headaches

1. **Generalized epilepsies:** Levetiracetam, topiramate, valproate, zonisamide
2. **Focal epilepsies:** Levetiracetam, topiramate, valproate, zonisamide.

References

Andermann E, Andermann FA. Migraine-epilepsy relationship: epidemiological and genetic aspects. In: Andermann FA, Lugaresi E, eds. *Migraine and Epilepsy* (pp. 281–291). Boston: Butterworths, 1987.

Ashkenazi A, Benlifer A, Korenblit J, Silberstein SD. Zonisamide for migraine prophylaxis in refractory patients. *Cephalalgia*. 2006;26: 1199–1202.

Aurora SK, Cao Y, Bowyer SM, et al. The occipital cortex is hyperexcitable in migraine: experimental evidence. *Headache*. 1999;39: 469–476.

Brandes JL, Saper JR, Diamond M, et al. Topiramate for migraine prevention: a randomized controlled trial. *Journal of the American Medical Association*. 2004;291: 965–973.

Buchanan TM, Ramadan NM. Prophylactic pharmacotherapy for migraine headaches. *Seminars in Neurology*. 2006;26: 188–198.

Calabresi P, Galletti F, Rossi C, Sarchielli P, Cupini LM. Antiepileptic drugs in migraine: from clinical aspects to cellular mechanisms. *Trends in Pharmacological Science,* 2007;28: 188–195.

D'Amico D. Antiepileptic drugs in the prophylaxis of migraine, chronic headache forms and cluster headache: a review of their efficacy and tolerability. *Neurological Sciences.* 2007;28: S188–S197.

de Tommaso M, Marinazzo D, Nitti L, Pellicoro M, Guido M, Serpino C, Stramaglia S. Effects of levetiracetam vs topiramate and placebo on visually evoked phase synchronization changes of alpha rhythm in migraine. *Clin Neurophysiol* 2007; 118(10): 2297–2304.

Diener HC, Bussone G, Van Oene JC, et al. Topiramate reduces headache days in chronic migraine: a randomized, double-blind, placebo-controlled study. *Cephalalgia.*2007;27: 814–823.

Freitag FG, Collins SD, Carlson HA, et al. A randomized trial of divalproex sodium extended-release tablets in migraine prophylaxis. *Neurology.* 2002;58: 1652–1659.

Koch UR, Musshoff U, Pannek HW, et al. Intrinsic excitability, synaptic potentials, and short-term plasticity in human epileptic neocortex. *Journal of Neuroscience Research.* 2005;80: 715–726.

Linde M, Mulleners WM, Chronicle EP, McCrory DC. Gabapentin or pregabalin for the prophylaxis of episodic migraine in adults. *Cochrane Database Syst Rev* 2013 Jun 24;6: CD010609.

Linde M, Mulleners WM, Chronicle EP, McCrory DC. Topiramate for the prophylaxis of episodic migraine in adults. *Cochrane Database Syst Rev* 2013 Jun 24; 6: CD010610.

Marks DA, Ehrenberg BL. Migraine related seizures in adults with epilepsy, with EEG correlation. *Neurology.* 1993; 43: 2476–2483.

Mathew NT, Rapoport A, Saper J, et al. Efficacy of gabapentin in migraine prophylaxis. *Headache.* 2001;41: 119–128.

Modi A, Lowder DM. Medications for migraine prophylaxis. *American Family Physician.* 2006;73: 72–78.

Mohammadianinejad SE, Abbasi V, Sajedi SA, Majdinasab N, Abdollahi F, Hajmanouchehri R, Faraji A. Zonisamide versus topiramate in migraine prophylaxis: a double-blind randomized clinical trial. *Clinical Neuropharmacology.* 2011;34(4): 174–177.

Ottman R, Lipton RB. Is the comorbidity of epilepsy and migraine due to a shared genetic susceptibility? *Neurology.* 1996;47: 918–924.

Palmieri A. Oxcarbazepine-induced headache. *Cephalalgia.* 2007;27: 91–93.

Pascual J, Lainez MJA, Dodick D, Hering-Hanit R. Antiepileptic drugs for the treatment of chronic and episodic cluster headache: a review. *Headache.* 2007;47: 81–89.

Pierangeli G, Cevoli S, Sancisi E, Grimaldi D, Zanigni S, Montagna P, Cortelli P. Which therapy for which patient? *Neurological Sciences.* 2006;27: S153–S158.

Steiner TJ, Findley LJ, Yuen AWC. Lamotrigine versus placebo in the prophylaxis of migraine with and without aura. *Cephalalgia.* 1997;17: 109–112.

Stevenson SB. Epilepsy and migraine headache: is there a connection? *Journal of Pediatric Health Care,* 2006;20: 167–171.

Chapter 25

Antiepileptic Drugs in Patients With Neuropathic Pain Syndromes

Neuropathic pain is defined as pain caused by dysfunction or a primary lesion in the central or peripheral nervous system. Examples of neuropathic pain syndromes include postherpetic neuralgia, painful diabetic neuropathy, central poststroke pain syndrome, trigeminal neuralgia, and HIV infection–associated neuralgia. Patients have described dull, throbbing, burning, or lancinating pain with these conditions (Vinik, 2005; Zaremba et al., 2006). These pains are often paroxysmal, especially trigeminal neuralgia. Neuropathic pain affects between 3% to 8% of the world's population, with unpleasant consequences on the patients' quality of life, general mood, and occupational functioning (Gilron & Coderre 2007; Bialer 2012).

Some antiepileptic drugs (AEDs) can suppress or attenuate pain in these conditions. It is assumed that both epilepsy and neuropathic pain share underlying common pathophysiology, enabling some AEDs to be useful for the treatment of several neuropathic pain conditions. Most AEDs reduce neuronal hyperexcitability by inhibiting ion channels, and they may act on different parts of the nociceptive pathway (Vinik, 2005; Bialer 2012). Carbamazepine was first approved for treatment of trigeminal neuralgia, years before approval was granted to treat epilepsy, and other agents have also found use in treating various neuropathic pain syndromes. Carbamazepine, gabapentin, and pregabalin are currently the only three AEDs approved for the treatment of neuropathic pain syndromes.

Carbamazepine

This drug is the most extensively investigated AED used in the management of trigeminal neuralgia. Carbamazepine often successfully treats trigeminal neuralgia and may at times help symptoms of painful diabetic neuropathy (Vinik, 2005; Maizels & McCarberg, 2005). However, efficacy may be limited over many years. One study evaluated the efficacy of carbamazepine over 16 years in 146 patients. The authors reported initial success in 60% of participants, but only 22% of participants still found carbamazepine effective by 5–16 years (Taylor et al., 1981).

Gabapentin

This AED is probably the best AED for the treatment of neuropathic pain, especially painful diabetic neuropathy and postherpetic neuralgia. Gabapentin should be used as one of the first-line drugs in painful diabetic neuropathy and postherpetic neuralgia even in patients without epilepsy (Serpel, 2002; Caraceni et al., 2004; Maizels and McCarberg, 2005; Wiffen et al., 2005; Vinik, 2005; Zaremba et al., 2006). While neither of these studies showed a dramatic overall improvement, worthwhile benefit was obtained by many patients.

Lacosamide

Lacosamide has limited efficacy in treating peripheral diabetic neuropathy with limited beneficial effect at higher doses. Results from various studies were of low quality, with moderate quality evidence for some efficacy outcomes of lacosamide (400 mg/day) (Bialer, 2012).

Lamotrigine

This agent has not been demonstrated as effective for neuropathic pain. While it has been advocated by some for the management of trigeminal neuralgia, painful diabetic neuropathy, HIV-associated neuropathy, and post-stroke pain syndrome (Maizels & McCarberg, 2005; Vinik, 2005; Zaremba et al., 2006), two randomized, double-blind, placebo-controlled studies were unable to demonstrate that lamotrigine was effective for pain associated with diabetic neuropathy (Vinik et al., 2007).

Oxcarbazepine

This AED has been reported to be effective in patients with trigeminal neuralgia, painful radiculopathy, and painful diabetic neuropathy (Zaremba et al., 2006; Beydoun et al., 2007; Jorns & Zakrzewska, 2007).

Phenytoin

This drug is useful in the treatment of trigeminal neuralgia (Zaremba et al., 2006).

Pregabalin

This drug is efficacious in the management of painful diabetic neuropathy and postherpetic neuralgia. In four clinical trials in a total of 1068 patients with diabetic peripheral neuropathy, patients receiving pregabalin at 300–600 mg/day had significantly greater improvement in mean pain scores than did placebo recipients. Patients with postherpetic neuralgia receiving pregabalin 450–600 mg/day had also significantly greater improvement in relief of pain and pain-related sleep interference than did placebo recipients (Maizels & McCarberg, 2005; Vinik, 2005; Zaremba et al., 2006; Tassone et al., 2007). How it compares with gabapentin is uncertain. Pregabalin treatment does not appear to be associated with loss of glycemic control. However, as the thiazolidinedione class of antidiabetic drugs can cause weight gain and/or fluid retention, possibly exacerbating or leading to heart failure, care should be taken when coadministering pregabalin and these agents in diabetic patients.

Valproate

Valproate is of uncertain efficacy for treating neuropathic pain syndromes (Vinik, 2005; Zaremba et al., 2006).

Topiramate

Topiramate may help painful diabetic neuropathy (Vinik, 2005), but it often causes unpleasant tingling in the fingers and toes, so it is not particularly desirable for the treatment of neuropathy.

Zonisamide

No satisfactory evidence exists at present supporting the use of zonisamide for the treatment of neuropathic pain (Krusz, 2003; Atli & Dogra, 2005).

In a recent systematic review for the treatment of painful diabetic neuropathy (PDN), pregabalin was ranked as the only level A drug for the relief of PDN. Gabapentin and valproate were considered as level B drugs for the treatment of PDN. Lacosamide, lamotrigine and oxcarbazepine were not recommended for PDN treatment (Brill et al., 2011). There are insufficient data in the literature to evaluate the role of the other AEDs, including phenobarbital, felbamate, tiagabine, and vigabatrin, in the treatment of neuropathic pain syndromes.

Recommended Antiepileptic Drugs in Epilepsy Patients With Neuropathic Pain Syndromes

1. **Generalized epilepsies:** Valproate
2. **Focal epilepsies:** Carbamazepine, gabapentin, pregabalin.

Note: Valproate, carbamazepine, gabapentin, and pregabalin may cause weight gain. Weight should be monitored in diabetic patients.

References

Atli A, Dogra S. Zonisamide in the treatment of painful diabetic neuropathy: a randomized, double-blind, placebo-controlled pilot study. *Pain Medicine*. 2005;6: 225–234.

Beydoun S, Alarcon F, Mangat S, Wan Y. Long-term safety and tolerability of oxcarbazepine in painful diabetic neuropathy. *Acta Neurologica Scandinavia*. 2007;115: 284–288.

Bialer M. Why are antiepileptic drugs used for nonepileptic conditions? *Epilepsia*. 2012; 53(Suppl. 7): 26–33.

Brill V, England J, Franklin GM, Backonja M, Choen J, Del R, Toro D, Feldman E, Iverson DJ, Perkins B, Russell JW, Zochodne D. Evidence-based guideline: treatment of painful diabetic neuropathy. *Neurology*. 2011;76: 1758–1765.

Caraceni A, Zecca E, Bonezzi C, et al. Gabapentin for neuropathic cancer pain: a randomized controlled trial from the Gabapentin Cancer Pain Study Group. *Journal of Clinical Oncology*. 2004;22: 2909–2917.

Gilron I, Coderre TJ. Emerging drugs in neuropathic pain. *Expert Opin Emerg Drugs*. 2007; 12: 113–126.

Jorns TP, Zakrzewska JM. Evidence-based approach to the medical management of trigeminal neuralgia. *British Journal of Neurosurgery*. 2007;21: 253–261.

Krusz JC. Treatment of chronic pain with zonisamide. *Pain Practice*. 2003;3: 317–320.

Maizels M, McCarberg B. Antidepressants and antiepileptic drugs for chronic non-cancer pain. *American Family Physician*. 2005;71: 483–490.

Serpell MG; Neuropathic Pain Study Group. Gabapentin in neuropathic pain syndromes: a randomised, double-blind, placebo-controlled trial. *Pain*. 2002;99: 557–566.

Tassone DM, Boyce E, Guyer J, Nuzum D. Pregabalin: a novel gamma aminobutiric acid analogue in the treatment of neuropathic pain, partial-onset seizures, and anxiety disorders. *Clinical Therapy*. 2007;29: 26–48.

Taylor, J. C., Brauer, S. and Espir, M LE. Long-term treatment of trigeminal neuralgia. *Postgraduate Medical Journal*. 1981;57: 16–18.

Vinik A. Use of antiepileptic drugs in the treatment of chronic painful diabetic neuropathy. *Journal of Clinical Endocrinology and Metabolism*. 2005;90: 4936–4945.

Vinik AI, Tuchman M, Safirstein B, et al. Lamotrigine for treatment of pain associated with diabetic neuropathy: results of two randomized, double-blind, placebo-controlled studies. *Pain*. 2007;128: 169–179.

Wiffen PJ, Mcquay HJ, Edwards JE, Moore RA. Gabapentin for acute and chronic pain. *Cochrane Database System Reviews*. 2005;3: CD005452.

Zaremba PD, Bialek M, Blaszczyk B, Cioczek P, Czuczwar SJ. Non-epilepsy uses of antiepileptic drugs. *Pharmacology Reports*. 2006;58: 1–12.

Chapter 26

Antiepileptic Drugs and Cutaneous/Allergic Reactions

Idiosyncratic drug reactions are unexpected and unpredictable adverse reactions, fundamentally different from the dose-related side effects of drugs. A variety of idiosyncratic reactions may occur, such as aplastic anemia, acute liver failure, and rash. Genetic factors may be important in many of these events (Pirmohamed & Park, 2001).

Drug-induced rashes are the most common type of idiosyncratic reaction due to the use of antiepileptic drugs (AEDs). The most common presentation is a maculopapular (Figure 26.1) or erythematous pruritic rash appearing within 4 weeks of initiating therapy with a new AED. Systemic symptoms are usually absent, although fever may occur. The rash usually disappears within several days of discontinuing the drug. Other therapeutic measures are rarely needed, although diphenhydramine may help suppress itching, and a brief course of steroids may be helpful for severe rash, particularly when fever is present. Occasionally, the rash can be severe and present as erythema multiforme, Stevens-Johnson syndrome, or toxic epidermal necrolysis (Lyell syndrome) (Asconapé, 2002; Alvestad et al., 2007).

The AED hypersensitivity syndrome (AHS), also known as drug reaction with eosinophilia and systemic symptoms (DRESS), is not common but is important and potentially life threatening. A triad of fever, skin rash, and internal organ involvement characterizes AHS. It usually starts within the first 2–8 weeks after initiation of therapy. The initial symptoms include a low-grade fever followed by rash, lymphadenopathy, and pharyngitis. This is followed by internal organ involvement (e.g., eosinophilia, hepatitis, and less commonly, nephritis, carditis, pneumonitis, myositis, or blood dyscrasias). Facial edema is a striking feature of AHS, particularly in the periorbital area (Figure 26.2). The reported rate of liver involvement ranges from 34% to 94%, and fulminant hepatic necrosis can be seen. The presence of hepatitis worsens prognosis. Prompt recognition is the mainstay of treatment of AHS. To establish whether a drug is the cause of an immune-mediated reaction such as AHS, alternative causes, latency of a reaction after drug intake, and improvement after drug cessation should be considered. The causative drug should be immediately discontinued. The patient should never be rechallenged with the offending agent, as the relapse rate is extremely high. Sometimes, even after discontinuation of the offending agent, the disease activity can persist for 2–16 weeks. Cross-reactivity among the aromatic AEDs may explain these prolonged symptoms after switching to another aromatic AED. The most controversial issue in the management of AHS is the use of systemic corticosteroids.

Figure 26.1 Generalized maculopapular rash on back.

Adapted from: Kocaoglu C, Cilasun C, Solak ES, Kurtipek GS, Arslan S. Successful treatment of antiepileptic drug-induced DRESS syndrome with pulse methylprednisolone. *Case Rep Pediatr.* 2013; 2013: 928910.

Although the role of corticosteroids is controversial, we advise prescribing prednisone, starting at a dosage of 1–2 mg/kg/day if symptoms are severe (e.g., hepatic involvement). Because stopping the offending AED increases the risk of having seizures, a new AED must be started immediately. In choosing a new drug, it is important to consider potential cross-reactivity and to try and avoid this problem. Valproate should be avoided if significant hepatic involvement has developed. Lacosamide, levetiracetam, gabapentin, pregabalin, and topiramate are reasonably safe options and can be immediately begun at therapeutic doses. Use of intermittent benzodiazepine therapy can help manage breakthrough seizure clusters during the transition. However, the structure of benzodiazepines contains aromatic rings, and part of their metabolism involves cytochrome P-450 isoforms. Therefore, there is still potential for cross-reactivity (Knowles et al., 1999; Asconapé, 2002; Kwong et al., 2006; Alvestad et al., 2007).

Stevens-Johnson and other severe syndromes have been reported in patients taking many AEDs. It is possible that lamotrigine is associated with a higher risk of developing a severe skin eruption than other drugs. Unfortunately, there is no reliable way to determine early in the clinical course of a rash if it will remain as a benign maculopapular rash or evolve into a severe skin reaction. Therefore, the offending drug should usually be discontinued as soon as possible. Signs and symptoms that may indicate the presence of a more severe reaction include a painful rash, mucosal involvement (Figure 26.3), fever, and other systemic symptoms (Asconapé, 2002).

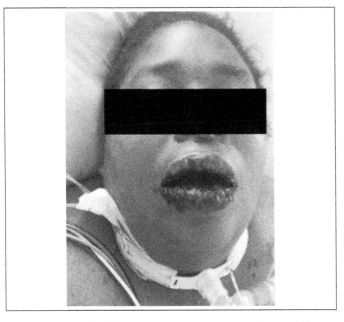

Figure 26.2 Severe facial edema in a patient with anticonvulsant hypersensitivity syndrome (AHS) or drug reaction with eosinophilia and systemic symptoms (DRESS).

Adapted from: Fleming P, Marik PE. The DRESS syndrome: the great clinical mimicker. *Pharmacotherapy* 2011;31(3): 45e-49e.

There are occasions, however, when it may be undesirable to stop a particular AED that has just caused a rash. In these circumstances, provided there are no signs of a more severe problem, one can continue that AED while observing the patient closely and treating symptoms such as itching with an antihistamine. Provided more severe symptoms do not appear, the rash will prove to be transient and disappear in many cases. This course of action should be carried out only when there are compelling reasons to continue an AED, or there is a strong presumption that the next drug will likely provoke a similar initial rash.

The aromatic (Figure 26.4) AEDs—phenytoin, carbamazepine, oxcarbazepine, eslicarbazepine acetate, phenobarbital, primidone, zonisamide, and lamotrigine—are more frequently associated with cutaneous eruptions and other signs or symptoms of drug hypersensitivity. There is a high degree of cross-reactivity (40%–80%) in patients with hypersensitivity or allergic reactions to phenytoin, phenobarbital, primidone, and carbamazepine. These drugs are all metabolized to hydroxylated aromatic compounds via the cytochrome P-450 hepatic enzymes. Arene oxide intermediates are formed during metabolism and are thought to be responsible for cross-sensitivity among these AEDs in susceptible individuals. Some individuals may have a reduced ability to detoxify intermediate toxic metabolites (e.g., arene oxides) of these

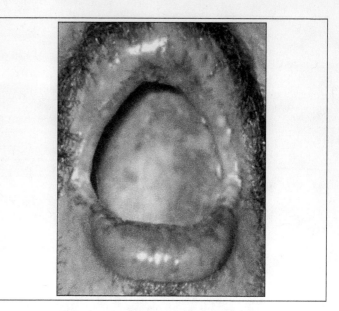

Figure 26.3 Multiple oral ulcers in a patient with Stevens-Johnson syndrome.

Adapted from: Reddy RB, Shekar PC, Chandra KL, Aravind R. Oral lesions associated with Nevirapine-induced Stevens-Johnson syndrome and toxic epidermal necrolysis: A report of 10 cases. *J Oral Maxillofac Pathol.* 2013;17(3): 431–435.

AEDs, which may be genetically mediated. However, there is no way to predict with certainty which patients will exhibit cross-sensitivity (Knowles et al., 1999; Asconapé, 2002; Levy et al., 2002; Kwong et al., 2006; Alvestad et al., 2007; *Drug Facts and Comparisons*, 2007). Whether drugs such as lamotrigine and zonisamide will also show a similar risk of cross-reactivity has not been

Figure 26.4 The aromatic chemical structure of eslicarbazepine acetate.

Adapted from: www.aptiom.com

properly evaluated, but it is likely due to the aromatic structure of these drugs. Nonaromatic AEDs (e.g., levetiracetam, topiramate, valproate) are safe alternatives for patients with aromatic AED-induced severe cutaneous adverse drug reactions.

According to a recent study, the rate of an AED rash is greater in patients with another AED rash (8.8%) versus in those without (1.7%) (odds ratio 3:1) (Arif et al., 2007). Therefore, patients with a history of an AED-induced rash should be treated with drugs with a lower risk for allergic reactions (e.g., valproate, benzodiazepines, gabapentin, topiramate, levetiracetam, or tiagabine). The rate of dose titration is also an important issue. The risk of allergic reaction is decreased when a drug is begun at a low dose and gradually increased; slow titration may allow desensitization to occur. A relation between starting dose and titration rate and the incidence of skin reactions is particularly evident for lamotrigine, carbamazepine, and phenytoin (Zaccara et al., 2007). Females may also be associated with a higher risk of AED-induced rash (Alvestad et al., 2007).

Skin testing, in particular the patch test, may be a useful screening method to discover the specific cause of an exanthematous cutaneous reaction if several drugs are possible offenders (Lammintausta & Kortekangas-Savolainen, 2005). In the unusual patient considered to be at high risk for a hypersensitivity reaction, skin tests to predict individual reactivity may be helpful (Zaccara et al., 2007).

Recent studies have shown that different ethnic populations may have dissimilar risks regarding the development of AED-severe cutaneous adverse drug reactions due to various genetic backgrounds. Genetic markers such as the human leukocyte antigen (HLA) are useful in predicting an individual's predisposition to AED hypersensitivity reactions. Ever since it was first linked with carbamazepine-SJS in Han Chinese, HLA allele B*1502 (HLA-B*1502) has become the strongest HLA correlation among human diseases. This association holds true for certain ethnic groups only, in particular Han Chinese, Thai, Malay, and to a lesser degree, Indians. Regardless of ethnicity, hypersensitivity reactions predisposition can be predicted by the in vitro lymphocyte toxicity assay (LTA) as well. LTA is a good predictor tool for possible hypersensitivity reactions in patients with epilepsy (Neuman et al., 2012).

Another potential adverse effect of AEDs is photosensitivity, which describes either a phototoxic response or a less frequent photoallergic reaction. A phototoxic reaction is immediate and resembles exaggerated sunburn. In comparison, a photoallergic reaction has an immunological basis and requires previous exposure to the photo-sensitizing agent. Patients who experience photoallergic responses typically present 1–14 days after exposure to sunlight with a papulovesicular eruption, pruritus, and eczematous dermatitis (Dubakiene & Kupriene, 2006). Photosensitivity reactions are not predictable and can occur at any age. Many medications, including antiepileptic drugs (AEDs), are associated with photosensitivity reactions (Moore, 2002; Dubakiene & Kupriene, 2006; *Drug Facts and Comparisons*, 2007). Protection from sunlight often prevents photosensitivity reactions. Avoidance of direct sunlight and sun-tanning facilities, using protective clothing and eyewear, application of an appropriate sunscreen with high UV protection rating, and evening dosing of the drug are measures that can minimize the risk of photosensitivity effects of most drugs (Moore, 2002; Dubakiene & Kupriene, 2006). Treatment is necessary when severe burning reaction occurs. In the case of a phototoxic reaction, the treatment is the same as used for sunburn. Avoidance of the offending photosensitizing agent or sunlight exposure is required, but sometimes an offending AED may not be avoidable. Therefore, preventive measures are of great significance. Antihistamines and corticosteroids may be required to treat the inflammation arising from photoallergic reactions (Moore, 2002). Should preventative measures be impractical or ineffective, then a new drug should be chosen. Photosensitivity has been reported with lamotrigine treatment in 2% of patients. Other AEDs associated with photosensitivity include carbamazepine, felbamate, gabapentin, oxcarbazepine, phenobarbital, phenytoin, tiagabine, topiramate, and valproic acid. The incidence of photosensitivity in patients taking these AEDs is less than 1%. Insufficient data are available for accurate estimates of incidence in most AEDs.

Note: Avoid lamotrigine and acetazolamide in patients with known photosensitivity to multiple drugs.

Acetazolamide

Acetazolamide is a sulfonamide. Acetazolamide has been associated with Stevens-Johnson syndrome, toxic epidermal necrolysis, and acute generalized exanthematous pustulosis. The nonfollicular, pustular, erythematous rash starts 2–3 weeks after starting the drug and is associated with fever. Reexposure may cause a second episode within 2 days. Acetazolamide is contraindicated in any patient with sulfonamide sensitivity (Levy et al., 2002; *Drug Facts and Comparisons,* 2007).

Like other sulfonamide derivatives, photosensitivity may occur with carbonic anhydrase inhibitors including acetazolamide. Some patients may be more sensitive to sunlight (UV) exposure while receiving acetazolamide.

Benzodiazepines

Drug-induced rashes and allergic reactions are not frequent with benzodiazepines (Levy et al., 2002; *Drug Facts and Comparisons,* 2007). Approximately 2% of patients taking clobazam develop a skin rash (Arif et al., 2007).

Carbamazepine

Some dermatological effects of carbamazepine include photosensitivity, alopecia, urticaria, alterations in skin pigmentation, exfoliative dermatitis, erythema multiforme, and erythema nodosum. Approximately 4%–11% of patients develop a skin rash (Alvestad et al., 2007; Arif et al., 2007). Rashes associated with carbamazepine do not have specific identifying characteristics.

The rash usually develops during the first 2–8 weeks of therapy. Serious dermatologic reactions including Stevens-Johnson syndrome, toxic epidermal necrolysis, and angioedema have been reported. Carbamazepine has also been associated with acute generalized exanthematous pustulosis. Multiorgan hypersensitivity reactions (AHS) occurring days to weeks or months after initiating treatment are rare (Levy et al., 2002; *Drug Facts and Comparisons,* 2007).

Eslicarbazepine Acetate

Serious dermatologic reactions including Stevens-Johnson syndrome (SJS) and also AHS have been reported in association with eslicarbazepine acetate. Rare cases of anaphylaxis and angioedema have been reported in patients taking this drug. Risk factors for development of these serious reactions have not been identified. This drug is chemically similar to carbamazepine and oxcarbazepine. Patients with a prior dermatologic reaction, AHS, or other serious reactions with either oxcarbazepine or eslicarbazepine acetate should not be treated with this drug.

Ethosuximide

Dermatological side effects during ethosuximide therapy include erythematous skin rash, pruritus, and urticaria. More serious reactions, which may be accompanied by fever, lymphadenopathy, pharyngitis, and muscle pain, are uncommon but can develop, including erythema multiforme and Stevens-Johnson syndrome. Ethosuximide should not be used in patients with a history of succinimide hypersensitivity (Levy et al., 2002; *Drug Facts and Comparisons,* 2007).

Ezogabine

Ezogabine can cause skin discoloration (blue, gray-blue, or brown). It is predominantly on or around the lips or in the nail beds of the fingers or toes, but more widespread involvement has also been reported. Approximately, 10% of patients in long-term clinical trials developed skin discoloration, generally after 2 or more years of treatment and at higher doses (900 mg or greater). Pathophysiology of skin discoloration with ezogabine remains unclear. The possibility of more extensive systemic involvement has not been excluded. If a patient develops skin discoloration, serious consideration should be given to changing to an alternate medication.

Felbamate

Acne, rash, and pruritus have occurred with felbamate therapy. Approximately 1%–2% of patients develop a skin rash (Arif et al., 2007). Toxic epidermal necrolysis due to felbamate has been reported. Felbamate is contraindicated in patients who have demonstrated hypersensitivity to the drug or its ingredients (Levy et al., 2002; *Drug Facts and Comparisons,* 2007).

Gabapentin

Less than 1% of patients develop a skin rash (Arif et al., 2007). Gabapentin is contraindicated in patients who have demonstrated hypersensitivity to the drug or its ingredients (Levy et al., 2002; *Drug Facts and Comparisons*, 2007).

Lacosamide

Mild (e.g., pruritus) and severe (e.g., AHS) reactions have been reported in patients taking lacosamide very rarely.

Lamotrigine

Rash is the most common cause for discontinuation of lamotrigine therapy. Approximately 10% of patients develop erythema and a maculopapular rash, although the incidence is lower when slow titration schedules are used (Arif et al., 2007). Rashes associated with lamotrigine do not have specific identifying characteristics. The rash usually develops during the first 2–8 weeks of therapy. Serious dermatological reactions including Stevens-Johnson syndrome, toxic epidermal necrolysis, and angioedema have been reported. Serious reactions are observed more often in children (8–10 in 1000) than adults (0.8–3 in 1000). Rash also appears to be more common in patients receiving valproic acid concomitantly or when the recommended dose escalation schedule is exceeded. The increased rate of rash observed in patients taking valproate when lamotrigine is initiated probably reflects reduced metabolism and therefore higher serum levels of lamotrigine (due to enzyme inhibition by valproate). Initiating therapy at the lowest possible dosage and escalating slowly appear to minimize the occurrence of skin rash. Bullous rash or vesicular rash should result in prompt discontinuation of lamotrigine therapy and appropriate evaluation. Hypersensitivity reactions, some fatal or life threatening, have also occurred with lamotrigine. Early manifestations of hypersensitivity (e.g., fever and lymphadenopathy) may be present even though a rash is not evident (Levy et al., 2002; Karande et al., 2006; *Drug Facts and Comparisons*, 2007).

Lamotrigine is contraindicated for use in any patient who has exhibited or is suspected of having hypersensitivity to lamotrigine or to any components of its formulation. Factors to predict a serious rash are not available; however, children appear to be at greater risk (Levy et al., 2002; *Drug Facts and Comparisons*, 2007), as are patients receiving valproate. In addition, a history of another AED-related rash is a major risk factor for developing rash to lamotrigine (Hirsch et al., 2006), and this drug should not be an early therapeutic choice for patients with a history of hypersensitivity to other AEDs.

Levetiracetam

Cutaneous eruptions rarely occur in patients treated with this drug (Arif et al., 2007). Levetiracetam is contraindicated in patients with a known hypersensitivity to the drug or any of the active ingredients in the formulations (Levy et al., 2002; *Drug Facts and Comparisons*, 2007).

Oxcarbazepine

Allergic skin reactions such as rash, pruritus, or urticaria may occur with oxcarbazepine. Approximately 2.5% of patients develop a skin rash (Arif et al., 2007). Rashes associated with oxcarbazepine do not have specific identifying characteristics. Other skin conditions reported include erythema multiforme and oral ulceration. Other serious dermatological reactions, including Stevens-Johnson syndrome and toxic epidermal necrolysis, have been reported in both children and adults in association with oxcarbazepine. AHS rarely occurs. Cross-sensitivity between carbamazepine and oxcarbazepine is approximately 25%–30% and is likely due to the structural similarity of the two drugs (Misra et al., 2003).

Oxcarbazepine should not be used in patients with a known hypersensitivity reaction to the drug or any of its components (Levy et al., 2002; *Drug Facts and Comparisons*, 2007).

Perampanel

No information is available with regard to potential dermatologic or allergic reactions with perampanel use.

Phenobarbital

Hypersensitivity reactions to phenobarbital may present as various organ system problems, including blood, liver, renal, and skin disorders. Discontinuation of the drug may not be sufficient to reverse progression of any serious hypersensitivity reaction because of the slow metabolism and excretion of phenobarbital.

Cutaneous reactions occur in 1%–2% of patients and include scarlatiniform or morbilliform maculopapular rash. Angioedema, bullous rash, exfoliative dermatitis, lupuslike symptoms, photosensitivity, purpura, serum sickness, Stevens-Johnson syndrome, and toxic epidermal necrolysis are rare but serious adverse effects of phenobarbital. Although uncommon, AHS has been reported with phenobarbital.

Avoid the use of phenobarbital in patients with a history of barbiturate hypersensitivity. Injectable solutions may also contain propylene glycol and should be avoided in patients with a hypersensitivity to propylene glycol. A history of hypersensitivity reactions should be obtained for a patient and the immediate family members. If hypersensitivity histories are positive, caution should be used in prescribing phenobarbital. Hypersensitivity reactions have been reported in patients who previously experienced phenytoin or carbamazepine hypersensitivity (Levy et al., 2002; *Drug Facts and Comparisons*, 2007). Patients who have experienced reactions due to phenobarbital therapy should not be further exposed to the drug.

Phenytoin

Adverse dermatological reactions to phenytoin occur in 5%–10% of patients and usually present as a maculopapular rash. More serious responses such as bullous rash, exfoliative dermatitis, purpura, erythema multiforme, Stevens-Johnson syndrome, or toxic epidermal necrolysis can occur but are rare. Minor reactions, such as rash, more often develop in the first few weeks of therapy in contrast to more serious reactions, which more often develop later. Skin hyperpigmentation has been reported and is more common in women than in men. Phenytoin can produce hypertrichosis or hirsutism. Coarsening of the facial features and enlargement of the lips are among the side effects.

Hypersensitivity reactions have been reported in patients who previously experienced other hydantoin hypersensitivity (e.g., fosphenytoin), barbiturate hypersensitivity (e.g., hypersensitivity to phenobarbital), or carbamazepine hypersensitivity (Levy et al., 2002; *Drug Facts and Comparisons*, 2007). Many patients who react to carbamazepine also react to phenytoin, and vice versa.

Pregabalin

The incidence of rash is low with this drug. Pregabalin is contraindicated in patients who have a demonstrated or suspected hypersensitivity to the drug or the inactive ingredients. It is not known if cross-hypersensitivity exists between gabapentin and pregabalin, but the drugs are chemically and structurally similar. Use pregabalin with caution in patients with a known hypersensitivity to gabapentin (Levy et al., 2002; *Drug Facts and Comparisons*, 2007).

Rufinamide

Rash, pruritus, Stevens-Johnson syndrome and AHS have rarely been reported in association with rufinamide therapy. All patients who develop a rash while taking rufinamide must be closely supervised. If any severe reaction (e.g., AHS) is suspected, rufinamide should be discontinued and alternative treatment started.

Tiagabine

Approximately 2.5% of patients develop a skin rash (Arif et al., 2007). Maculopapular rash, vesicular rash, and (in rare cases) Stevens-Johnson syndrome have been reported due to tiagabine (Levy et al., 2002; *Drug Facts and Comparisons*, 2007).

Topiramate

Approximately 1% of patients develop a rash (Arif et al., 2007). Topiramate is contraindicated in any patient hypersensitive to the drug or any of the product components. Rarely, serious and potentially fatal exfoliative dermatologic reactions have been reported (Levy et al., 2002; *Drug Facts and Comparisons*, 2007).

Valproic Acid

Dermatological reactions have been seen in patients receiving valproic acid. These reactions include transient alopecia, skin rash, pruritus, photosensitivity, erythema multiforme, and Stevens-Johnson syndrome (Levy et al., 2002; *Drug Facts and Comparisons*, 2007). Approximately 1% of patients develop a rash (Arif et al., 2007). Multiorgan hypersensitivity reactions (AHS) have been rarely reported with valproate. Cross-sensitivity with other drugs that produce this syndrome is unclear but may be possible (Levy et al., 2002; *Drug Facts and Comparisons*, 2007). As noted, patients taking valproate are more likely to develop a rash when lamotrigine is begun.

Vigabatrin

Angioedema, maculo-papular rash, pruritus, Stevens-Johnson syndrome, and toxic epidermal necrolysis (TEN) have been reported by patients taking vigabatrin.

Zonisamide

Approximately 4.5% of patients develop a rash (Arif et al., 2007). Zonisamide is a sulfonamide and can, in rare cases, produce severe, possibly fatal reactions such as toxic epidermal necrolysis, Stevens-Johnson syndrome, fulminant hepatic necrosis, and blood dyscrasias. Once sensitization to sulfonamides has occurred, a recurrence can be precipitated by administration of sulfonamides by any route. Zonisamide should be discontinued if there is any sign of a hypersensitivity reaction. Rash usually develops early (2–16 weeks) in the course of treatment with zonisamide.

Zonisamide is more likely to cause rash in patients with a history of sulfonamide hypersensitivity. Additionally, zonisamide should be avoided if possible in patients with carbonic anhydrase inhibitor hypersensitivity (Levy et al., 2002; *Drug Facts and Comparisons*, 2007).

Recommended Antiepileptic Drugs in Patients With History of Drug-Induced Skin Rash

1. **Generalized epilepsies:** Levetiracetam, topiramate, valproate
2. **Focal epilepsies:** Gabapentin, lacosamide, levetiracetam, perampanel, pregabalin, topiramate.

Note: The risk for cutaneous adverse effects (e.g., Stevens-Johnson syndrome and toxic epidermal necrolysis) with phenytoin, phenobarbital, and carbamazepine is increased during radiotherapy. When treatment is indicated, a drug with a lower potential for allergic cutaneous reactions (e.g., gabapentin, levetiracetam, pregabalin, or topiramate) is preferred (Michelucci, 2006).

References

Alvestad S, Lydersen S, Brodtkorb E. Rash from antiepileptic drugs: influence by gender, age, and learning disability. *Epilepsia*. 2007;48: 1360–1365.

Arif H, Buchsbaum R, Weintraub D, et al. Comparisons and predictors of rash associated with 15 antiepileptic drugs. *Neurology*. 2007;68: 1701–1709.

Asconapé JJ. Some common issues in the use of antiepileptic drugs. *Seminars in Neurology*. 2002;22: 27–39.

Drug Facts and Comparisons. St. Louis: Wolters Kluwer Health/Facts & Comparisons, 2007.

Dubakiene R, Kupriene M. Scientific problems of photosensitivity. *Medicina*. 2006;42: 619–628.

Fleming P, Marik PE. The DRESS syndrome: the great clinical mimicker. *Pharmacotherapy*. 2011;31(3): 45e–49e.

Hirsch LJ, Weintraub DB, Buchsbaum R, Spencer HT, Straka T, Hager M, Resor SR Jr. Predictors of lamotrigine-associated rash. *Epilepsia*. 2006;47: 318–322.

Karande S, Gogtay NJ, Kanchan S, Kshirsagar NA. Anticonvulsant hypersensitivity syndrome to lamotrigine confirmed by lymphocyte stimulation in vitro. *Indian Journal of Medical Sciences*. 2006;60: 59–63.

Knowles SR, Shapiro LE, Shear NH. Anticonvulsant hypersensitivity syndrome: incidence, prevention and management. *Drug Safety*. 1999;21: 489–501.

Kocaoglu C, Cilasun C, Solak ES, Kurtipek GS, Arslan S. Successful treatment of antiepileptic drug-induced DRESS syndrome with pulse methylprednisolone. *Case Rep Pediatr* 2013; 928910.

Kwong KL, Lam SY, Lui YS, Wong SN, So KT. Cross-sensitivity in a child with anticonvulsant hypersensitivity syndrome. *Journal of Paediatrics and Child Health*. 2006;42: 474–476.

Lammintausta K, Kortekangas-Savolainen O. The usefulness of skin tests to prove drug hypersensitivity. *British Journal of Dermatology*. 2005;152: 968–974.

Levy RH, Mattson RH, Meldrum BS, Perucca E. *Antiepileptic Drugs*. 5th ed. Philadelphia: Lippincott Williams & Wilkins, 2002.

Michelucci R. Optimizing therapy of seizures in neurosurgery. *Neurology*. 2006;67: S14–S18.

Misra UK, Kalita J, Rathore C. Phenytoin and carbamazepine cross reactivity: report of a case and review of literature. *Postgraduate Medical Journal*. 2003;79: 703–704.

Moore DE. Drug-induced cutaneous photosensitivity. *Drug Safety*. 2002;25: 345–372.

Neuman MG, Cohen L, Nanau RM, Hwang PA. Genetic and immune predictors for hypersensitivity syndrome to antiepileptic drugs. *Transl Res* 2012;159(5): 397–406.

Pirmohamed M, Park BK. Genetic susceptibility to adverse drug reactions. *Trends in Pharmacological Science*. 2001;22: 298–305.

Reddy RB, Shekar PC, Chandra KL, Aravind R. Oral lesions associated with Nevirapine-induced Stevens-Johnson syndrome and toxic epidermal necrolysis: A report of 10 cases. *J Oral Maxillofac Pathol* 2013;17(3): 431–435.

Zaccara G, Franciotta D, Perucca E. Idiosyncratic adverse reactions to antiepileptic drugs. *Epilepsia*. 2007;48: 1223–1244.

Sunovion. http://www.aptiom.com/2014

Eisai. http://www.banzel.com/2014

GSK. http://www.potiga.com/2014

UCB. http://www.vimpat.com/2014

Eisai. http://www.fycompa.com/2014

Lundbeck. http://www.sabril.net/2014

Chapter 27

Antiepileptic Drugs and Ophthalmologic Problems

Ophthalmologic problems in patients with epilepsy may be due to either the disease process or therapy with antiepileptic drugs (AEDs). Visual disturbances such as blurred vision, diplopia, and oscillopsia are generally benign, reversible, dose-dependent neurotoxic side effects of AEDs (Table 27.1). The dose of medication simply needs to be reduced or the dosing frequency increased to abolish this complaint in most instances. However, some patients have visual complaints at relatively low serum levels, and the offending AED must be stopped and replaced with another.

Other ocular complaints may be related to the unique mechanistic properties of the drug and can occur when they are administered at therapeutic levels. This is true of vigabatrin and ezogabine, which have special retinal toxicity that has greatly limited their use.

Ezogabine

Ezogabine can cause abnormalities of the retina. These abnormalities have funduscopic features similar to those seen in retinal pigment dystrophies that are known to result in damage to photoreceptors and vision loss. Approximately, one-third of the patients who had ophthalmologic examinations performed after 4 years of treatment were found to have retinal pigmentary abnormalities. Funduscopic abnormalities have most commonly been described as perivascular pigmentation (bone spicule pattern) in the retinal periphery and/or as areas of focal retinal pigment epithelium clumping. The rate of progression of retinal abnormalities and the reversibility after drug discontinuation are unknown.

Because of the observed ophthalmologic adverse reactions, ezogabine should only be used in patients who have responded inadequately to several alternative AEDs and for whom the benefits outweigh the risks. Patients who fail to show substantial clinical benefit after adequate titration should be discontinued from ezogabine. Patients should have baseline ophthalmologic testing and follow-up testing every 6 months. The ophthalmologic monitoring program should include visual acuity testing and dilated fundus photography. Additional testing may include fluorescein angiograms (FA), ocular coherence tomography (OCT), perimetry, and electroretinograms (ERG). If retinal pigmentary abnormalities or vision changes are detected, ezogabine should be discontinued unless no other suitable treatment options are available and the benefits of treatment outweigh the potential risk of vision loss.

Table 27.1 Visual Adverse Effects of Antiepileptic Drugs

Antiepileptic Drug	Visual Adverse Effects
Acetazolamide	Enhanced ocular blood flow, decreased intra-ocular pressure
Benzodiazepine	Blurred vision, visual electrophysiological changes, maculopathy
Carbamazepine	Blurred vision, diplopia, abnormal color perception, nystagmus, oscillopsia (illusionary movements of objects), altered visual evoked potentials (VEPs), ophthalmoplegia
Eslicarbazepine acetate	Diplopia, blurred vision, impaired vision, nystagmus
Ethosuximide	Photophobia, myopia
Ezogabine	Retinal pigmentary abnormalities, blurred vision, diplopia, nystagmus
Felbamate	Blurred vision, diplopia, miosis, hemianopia, conjunctivitis
Gabapentin	Amblyopia, blurred vision, nystagmus, diplopia, visual electrophysiological changes, impaired critical flicker frequency
Lacosamide	Diplopia, blurred vision, nystagmus
Lamotrigine	Blurred vision, diplopia, visual electrophysiological disturbances, nystagmus
Levetiracetam	Blurred vision, diplopia
Oxcarbazepine	Diplopia, blurred vision
Perampanel	Diplopia, blurred vision
Phenobarbital	Blurred vision, miosis, mydriasis, ophthalmoplegia
Phenytoin	Nystagmus, ophthalmoplegia, blurred vision, diplopia, disturbed color perception
Pregabalin	Blurred vision, diplopia, nystagmus, conjunctivitis
Primidone	Blurred vision, diplopia, nystagmus, ophthalmoplegia
Rufinamide	Diplopia, blurred vision, nystagmus
Tiagabine	Abnormal color perception, blurred vision, nystagmus, diplopia
Topiramate	Blurred vision, diplopia, acute myopia, acute angle closure glaucoma, suprachoroidal effusions, nystagmus, conjunctivitis
Valproate	Abnormal color perception, altered VEPs, blurred vision, diplopia, nystagmus
Vigabatrin	Diplopia, nystagmus, peripheral visual field loss, color perception abnormalities, retinal abnormalities, optic nerve pallor, visual electrophysiological changes, reduced contrast sensitivity, reduced ocular blood flow
Zonisamide	Blurred vision, diplopia, nystagmus

Vigabatrin

A drug that acts on the GABAergic pathway, vigabatrin causes a visual disturbance (Hilton et al., 2004; Bhattacharyya & Basu, 2005). This is due to the concentration of this drug in retinal glial cells that results in toxicity, ultimately affecting foveal and peripheral cone cells. Other AEDs that act on GABAergic pathways do not accumulate in the retina to the same extent as vigabatrin and do not have retinal toxicity.

The onset of vision loss from vigabatrin is unpredictable and can occur at any time after starting treatment. Symptoms of vision loss from vigabatrin are unlikely to be recognized by patients or caregivers before vision loss is severe. Vigabatrin-associated visual disturbances can be identified with electroretinograms and visual field perimetry. Perimetry defects characteristically present as bilateral concentric nasal constriction with temporal and central sparing, a pattern rarely seen in other conditions. Approximately, 30% (20%–50%) of epilepsy patients receiving the drug at normal therapeutic doses have visual field abnormalities (You et al., 2006). Men receiving vigabatrin are more susceptible to visual field constriction than are women, and adults are probably more susceptible than are children. The vast majority of patients with vigabatrin-associated visual field constriction are asymptomatic. In clinical practice, patients with visual field defects often remain asymptomatic until the defect impinges on, or is close to, fixation; this is particularly likely in the case of binasal defects where the preserved temporal visual field in each eye enables patients to retain good mobility. Longitudinal investigations of vigabatrin-associated visual field loss have reported the defects to be permanent, persisting even after patients are withdrawn from the drug (Hilton et al., 2004). However, visual field defects were found to be reversible in two children treated with vigabatrin when the drug was withdrawn (Nabbout, 2001).

For this reason, vigabatrin is reserved for situations when no other drug offers hope or when a short-term course of therapy is planned. For children with tuberous sclerosis who have infantile spasms, the benefits of vigabatrin monotherapy appear to outweigh the risks (Nabbout, 2001; Hilton et al., 2004; You et al., 2006). It is not clear that other conditions warrant the use of this agent. When treatment with vigabatrin is indicated, visual field testing (e.g., perimetry) should be carried out at the start of treatment (within 4 weeks of the start of treatment) and at regular time intervals (every 3 months); electroretinography may help detect abnormalities as well, perhaps before field loss appears (Figure 27.1). Finally, vigabatrin should be withdrawn from patients with refractory complex partial seizures within 3 months of initiation and within 2 to 4 weeks of initiation for patients with infantile spasms, who fail to show substantial clinical benefit.

Because of the risk of permanent vision loss, vigabatrin is available only through a restricted program under a Risk Evaluation and Mitigation Strategy (REMS) called the Support, Help and Resources for Epilepsy (SHARE) program.

Figure 27.1 Recommended screening algorithm for patients with (a) complex partial seizures and (b) infantile spasms, taking vigabatrin.

ERG: Electroretinography; OCT: Optical coherence tomography; VGB: Vigabatrin; pVFD: Peripheral visual field defect.

Adapted from: Sergott RC, Wheless JW, Smith MC, Westall CA, Kardon RH, Arnold A, Foroozan R, Sagar SM. Evidence-based review of recommendations for visual function testing in patients treated with Vigabatrin. *Neuro-Ophthalmology* 2010;34(1): 20–35.

Other Antiepileptic Drugs

Ocular pathology is rarely provoked by topiramate. This drug can cause acute myopia and secondary closed angle glaucoma without pupillary block. These findings are more common in females, occur when serum levels are within a normal therapeutic range, and usually appear within the first month of therapy. The symptoms include an acute onset of decreased visual acuity and/or ocular pain. Ophthalmologic examination may reveal myopia, ocular hyperemia, shallowing of the anterior chamber, and elevated intraocular pressure, with or without pupil dilation; choroidal effusions have also been described. It has been suggested that supraciliary effusion and ciliary body swelling may displace the lens and iris anteriorly, secondarily resulting in angle closure glaucoma (Hilton et al., 2004; Bhattacharyya & Basu, 2005).

Benzodiazepines are reportedly contraindicated in patients with acute closed-angle glaucoma according to recommendations of official drug information materials. However, a systematic review of the literature reveals that this contraindication is based on only one published case, while 22 other investigations, some of them controlled, found that benzodiazepines reduce intraocular pressure (Fritze et al., 2002). Hence, this recommendation is probably not valid, and benzodiazepines may be used in patients with glaucoma.

Ophthalmoplegia has been reported consequent to administration of phenytoin, phenobarbital, primidone, and carbamazepine. Phenytoin can induce external ophthalmoplegia whether administered orally or intravenously. Incomplete as well as complete ophthalmoplegia has been reported with phenytoin even within therapeutic range (Fredericks et al., 1986; Spector and Davidoff, 1976; Puri and Chaudhry, 2004; Drugs' websites).

References

Bhattacharyya KB, Basu S. Acute myopia induced by topiramate: report of a case and review of the literature. *Neurology India*. 2005;53: 108–109.

Drug Facts and Comparisons. St. Louis: Wolters Kluwer Health/Facts & Comparisons, 2007.

Fredericks CA, Giannotta SL, Sadun AA. Dilantin-induced long-term bilateral total external ophthalmoplegia. *Clinical Neuro-ophthalmology*. 1986;6: 22–26.

Fritze J, Schneider B, Weber B. Benzodiazepines and benzodiazepine-like anxiolytics and hypnotics: the implausible contraindication of angle-closure glaucoma. *Nervenartz*. 2002;73: 50–53.

Hilton EJR, Hosking SL, Betts T. The effect of antiepileptic drugs on visual performance. *Seizure*. 2004;13: 113–128.

Nabbout R. A risk-benefit assessment of treatment for infantile spasms. *Drug Safety*. 2001;24: 813–828.

Puri V, Chaudhry N. Total external ophthalmoplegia induced by phenytoin: a case report and review of literature. *Neurology India*. 2004;52: 386–387.

Sergott RC, Wheless JW, Smith MC, Westall CA, Kardon RH, Arnold A, Foroozan R, Sagar SM. Evidence-based review of recommendations for visual function testing in patients treated with Vigabatrin. *Neuro-Ophthalmology*. 2010; 34(1): 20–35.

Spector RH, Davidoff RA, Schwartzman RJ. Phenytoin-induced ophthalmoplegia. *Neurology*. 1976;26: 1031.

You SJ, Ahn HS, Ko TS. Vigabatrin and visual field defects in pediatric epilepsy patients. *Journal of Korean Medical Science*. 2006;21: 728–732.

Sunovion. http://www.aptiom.com/2014

Eisai. http://www.banzel.com/2014

GSK. http://www.potiga.com/2014

UCB. http://www.vimpat.com/2014

Eisai. http://www.fycompa.com/2014

Lundbeck. http://www.sabril.net/2014

Chapter 28

Antiepileptic Drugs and Weight Change

Many patients experience weight change after starting an antiepileptic drug (AED). Some AEDs are associated with weight loss, some with weight gain, and others have no effect. Weight gain is associated with an increased risk of comorbidities (e.g., type 2 diabetes, mellitus, and heart diseases) and impairs quality of life and self-esteem. Weight loss is also associated with comorbidity (e.g., osteoporosis, immune, and metabolic problems) (Pickrell et al., 2013). Depending on comorbid conditions (i.e., chiefly obesity, diabetes, and, at times, poor appetite) one might consider choosing an AED that may influence weight in a positive way. For example, an obese patient, particularly one who is diabetic, might secondarily benefit by taking an AED that causes weight loss (e.g., topiramate). A patient with poor appetite who is underweight might profit by taking an AED that causes weight gain. Avoidance of drugs that cause weight gain might be important to many patients and their physicians. In any case, one must have knowledge of this AED side effect and consider that it can be used to advantage in selected patients.

The treating physician should adequately explain risks of weight change with AEDs to patients; if not then they may lose the opportunity to ameliorate the risk via prospectively monitoring their weight and executing early lifestyle changes. Besides, subsequent weight change may contribute to discontinuation of the associated AED (Pickrell et al., 2013). Box 28.1 summarizes the effects of the various AEDs on weight and might therefore be used as a guide.

Carbamazepine

Weight gain has been reported in 2%–25% of patients during carbamazepine therapy. This wide range suggests that the true incidence is not known. In the experience of the authors, significant weight gain is rare. Weight gain with carbamazepine could be related to water retention; however, increased appetite and increase in weight without edema have also been described (Jallon & Picard, 2001).

Eslicarbazepine Acetate

No significant weight changes have been reported in patients taking this drug.

Box 28.1 Antiepileptic Drugs and Weight Change

Weight Gain	Weight Loss	No Effect on Weight	Not Defined
Valproate	Topiramate	Phenytoin	Phenobarbital
Pregabalin	Zonisamide	Lamotrigine	Ethosuximide
Gabapentin	Felbamate	Levetiracetam (?)	—
Vigabatrin	Acetazolamide (?)	Oxcarbazepine	—
Carbamazepine	Rufinamide	Tiagabine	—
Ezogabine	—	Eslicarbazepine	—
Perampanel	—	Lacosamide	—

From Futagi et al. (1996), Hogan et al. (2000), Jallon and Picard (2001), Asconapé (2002), Biton (2006), and Connor et al. (2006), drug's websites.

Ethosuximide

There is no evidence that ethosuximide affects weight.

Ezogabine

Ezogabine was associated with dose-related weight gain.

Felbamate

In clinical trials with felbamate, anorexia and weight loss were among the most common adverse events. Anorexia was reported in approximately 10–20% of patients; weight loss, which can be transient, is reported in up to 3%–6% of patients. Weight loss with felbamate varies in severity. Among those older than 15 years, mean weight loss was almost 4% of the baseline weight. The mechanism by which felbamate affects weight is unknown. Patients who lose weight with felbamate nearly always report anorexia; therefore, reduction in caloric intake may be responsible for the reduction in weight (Biton, 2003).

Gabapentin

Weight gain up to more than 10% of the baseline weight during gabapentin therapy has been reported in about 6% of patients. The mechanisms of bodyweight gain with gabapentin could reflect the enhancement of GABA-mediated inhibition in the medial hypothalamus (Jallon & Picard, 2001). Weight loss associated with anorexia has rarely been reported in some patients.

Lacosamide

No significant weight changes have been reported in patients taking this drug.

Lamotrigine

No significant weight changes have been reported in patients taking this drug.

Levetiracetam

No significant weight changes have been reported in patients taking this drug in most studies. One recent study reported significant weight gain associated with levetiracetam (Pickrell et al., 2013).

Oxcarbazepine

Weight gain or weight loss has infrequently been reported.

Perampanel

Perampanel-treated adults gained an average of 1.1 kg (2.5 lbs) compared to an average of 0.3 kg (0.7 lbs) in placebo-treated adults. The percentages of adults who gained at least 7% and 15% of their baseline body weight in perampanel-treated patients were 9.1% and 0.9%, respectively.

Phenobarbital

The effects of phenobarbital on weight change have not been studied well. No systematic changes have been observed.

Phenytoin

Phenytoin does not have significant effects on weight.

Pregabalin

Since the time pregabalin became available for routine clinical use, reports of weight gain associated with its use have been published. Preclinical trials suggest significant weight gain (> 7%) in 15%–20% of subjects, depending upon dose (Elger et al., 2005).

Rufinamide

Decreased weight has been reported in patients receiving rufinamide both in the presence and absence of gastrointestinal symptoms.

Tiagabine

Weight gain was observed in 2% of patients taking tiagabine in preclinical trials, which is probably not significant (Cephalon, Inc., n.d.).

Topiramate

Topiramate has been shown to have hypothalamic effects, which could explain the reduction in appetite (Eliasson et al., 2007). The anorectic effect of topiramate may be due to its antagonism of glutamate (Ioannides-Demos et al., 2005). Patients treated with topiramate experienced mean percent reductions in weight that were dose dependent. Nine percent of patients taking 200–400 mg/day and up to 13% of patients receiving doses above 600 mg/day will experience weight loss. Weight loss is highest in patients with a high body mass index (Biton, 2003).

Valproate

As many as 50% of patients taking valproate experience weight gain (Isojarvi et al., 1996). The magnitude of weight gain varied substantially between studies from approximately 5 to 50 kg. Lowered blood glucose level has been proposed as one mechanism that could lead to obesity with valproate therapy. As an alternative hypothesis, valproate may increase appetite for carbohydrates and reduce energy expenditure by enhancing GABA-mediated neurotransmission. It is not clear that whether this effect is dose dependent. Rarely, anorexia with weight loss has been reported in patients taking this drug (Jallon & Picard, 2001; Biton, 2003).

Vigabatrin

As many as 47% of patients taking vigabatrin experience weight gain. Weight gain is not related to the occurrence of edema.

Zonisamide

More than one-quarter of patients taking zonisamide lost more than 5 lbs in one study. Zonisamide displays dose-dependent serotonergic and dopaminergic activities that may contribute to its anorectic effect (Gadde et al., 2003; Ioannides-Demos et al., 2005).

Recommended Antiepileptic Drugs in Obese Patients With Epilepsy

1. **Generalized epilepsies:** Lamotrigine, rufinamide (in patients with Lennox-Gastaut syndrome), topiramate, zonisamide
2. **Focal epilepsies:** Eslicarbazepine acetate, lacosamide, lamotrigine, phenytoin, topiramate, zonisamide

References

Asconapé JJ. Some common issues in the use of antiepileptic drugs. *Seminars in Neurology*. 2002;22: 27–39.

Biton V. Effect of antiepileptic drugs on bodyweight: overview and clinical implications for the treatment of epilepsy. *CNS Drugs*. 2003;17: 781–791.

Biton V. Weight change and antiepileptic drugs. *The Neurologist*. 2006;10: 163–167.

Cephalon, Inc. *Gabitril*. Retrieved from http://www.gabitril.com/download/148–3230 EnlargedPI.pdf.

Connor KM, Davidson JRT, Weisler RH, Zhang W, Abraham K. Tiagabine for post-traumatic stress disorder: effect of open-label and double-blind discontinuation treatment. *Psychopharmacology*. 2006;184: 21–25.

Elger CE, Brodie MJ, Anhut J, Lee CM, Barrett JA. Pregabalin add-on treatment in patients with partial seizures: a novel evaluation of flexible-dose and fixed-dose treatment in a double-blind, placebo-controlled study. *Epilepsia*. 2005;46: 1926–1936.

Eliasson B, Gudbjornsdottir S, Cederholm J, Liang Y, Vercruysse F, Smith U. Weight loss and metabolic effects of topiramate in overweight and obese type 2 diabetic patients: randomized double-blind placebo-controlled trial. *International Journal of Obesity*. 2007;31: 1140–1147.

Futagi Y, Otani K, Abe J. Growth suppression in children receiving acetazolamide with antiepileptic drugs. *Pediatric Neurology*. 1996;15: 323–326.

Gadde KM, Franciscy DM, Wagner HR, et al. Zonisamide for weight loss in obese adults. *Journal of American Medical Association*. 2003;289: 1820–1825.

Hogan RE, Bertrand ME, Deaton RL, Sommerville KW. Total percentage body weight changes during add-on therapy with tiagabine, carbamazepine and phenytoin. *Epilepsy Research*. 2000;41: 23–28.

Ioannides-Demos LL, Proietto J, McNeil JJ. Pharmacotherapy for obesity. *Drugs*. 2005;65: 1391–1418.

Isojarvi JI, Laatikainen TJ, Knip M, Pakarinen AJ, Juntunen KT, Myllyla VV. Obesity and endocrine disorders in women taking valproate for epilepsy. *Annals of Neurology*. 1996;39: 579–584.

Jallon P, Picard F. Bodyweight gain and anticonvulsants: a comparative review. *Drug Safety*. 2001;24: 969–978.

Pickrell WO, Lacey AS, Thomas RH, Smith PE, Rees MI. Weight change associated with antiepileptic drugs. *J Neurol Neurosurg Psychiatry* 2013; 84(7): 796–799.

Janssen Pharm. Inc. http://www.topamax.com/topamax/assets/topamax.pdf/2012.

Sunovion. http://www.aptiom.com/2014
Eisai. http://www.banzel.com/2014
GSK. http://www.potiga.com/2014
UCB. http://www.vimpat.com/2014
Eisai. http://www.fycompa.com/2014
Lundbeck. http://www.sabril.net/2014

Chapter 29

Antiepileptic Drugs and Bone Health

Patients taking antiepileptic drugs (AEDs) have higher rates of osteopenia, osteoporosis, and bone fractures than the general population (Gissel et al., 2007; Beniczky et al., 2012). Good population-based epidemiological studies are rare, but published studies evaluating bone density in patients recruited from epilepsy clinics suggest that the rate of osteopenia and osteoporosis generally is 40%–75%, and the magnitude of the reduction in real bone mineral density may be as high as 16% (Petty et al., 2005); although other studies have found varying percentages, all have found a relatively high prevalence of bone demineralization in people with epilepsy. Decrease in bone mineral density leads to increased bone fragility and, hence, greater risk of fracture. When one considers that people with epilepsy have a greater propensity for falls as well, the reduction in bone density has even greater importance than usual.

There are probably multiple causes of the increased rate of osteopenia and osteoporosis in epilepsy. They may be caused in part by effects of the disease on lifestyle and income. People with epilepsy may have reduced activity levels compared with the general population and tend to have lower incomes, which might impact dietary habits. However, AEDs probably cause reduced bone density by virtue of their metabolic effects. Most of the available data describe bone density and metabolism in patients taking older AEDs (phenytoin, phenobarbital, carbamazepine, and valproate), although information is becoming available about some of the newer AEDs (Mintzer et al., 2006; Beniczky et al., 2012). This chapter will briefly review how AEDs can produce bone demineralization and how this might be prevented.

Evidence suggests that AEDs may have negative effects on bone mineral density through a variety of mechanisms (Ali et al., 2004). Decrease in bone mineral density is thought to be related to decreased intestinal absorption of calcium, accelerated vitamin-D hydroxylation to inactive forms, increased bone turnover, impairment of PTH (parathyroid hormone)-induced calcium mobilization, interference with vitamin-K metabolism, inhibition of osteocalcin, increased urinary loss of calcium and phosphorus due to renal tubular dysfunction, and probably other reasons. There is an extensive body of literature that suggests that AEDs can produce hypocalcemia, hypophosphatemia, increased alkaline phosphatase levels, a slight increase in the parathormone level, and a decrease in biologically active vitamin-D levels.

Many of the above-cited effects can be attributed to induction of the cytochrome P-450 system enzymes. Carbamazepine, phenytoin, phenobarbital, and primidone, all enzyme inducers, increase the metabolism of vitamin D and its active metabolite, lowering their serum levels. Decreased vitamin-D levels may result in decreased calcium absorption, secondary hyperparathyroidism, and decrease in bone density (Babayigit et al., 2006). One of the newer AEDs, oxcarbazepine, also significantly reduces 25-hydroxy vitamin-D levels and increases bone-specific alkaline phosphatase, which is a marker of bone formation (Mintzer et al., 2006). The effects of AEDs may be additive (when used as polytherapy) (Farhat et al., 2002; Shen et al., 2014). While the theoretical basis for enzyme-inducing AEDs causing decreased bone density seems relatively strong, the association of valproate, a cytochrome P-450 inhibitor (Babayigit et al., 2006; Gissell et al., 2007), and non-enzyme-inducing AEDs (e.g., gabapentin) with osteoporosis raises the possibility that a more complex picture exists (Ensrud et al., 2008; Shen et al., 2014). No convincing rationales exist to explain this association. Some data suggest that lamotrigine may not have a deleterious effect on metabolic indices of bone turnover (Pack et al., 2005; Sheth & Hermann, 2007). Data regarding the effects of levetiracetam and oxcarbazepine on bone health in human and animal studies are conflicting (Beniczky et al., 2012; Fekete et al., 2013; Koo et al., 2013; Koo et al., 2014). Data regarding the effects of the newer AEDs (e.g., lacosamide, perampanel, etc.) on bone health is not available yet.

What advice can a physician offer patients who take AEDs? Box 29.1 summarizes recommendations for patient care.

Given the tendency of many AEDs to produce bone loss, measurement of bone density may be useful during the course of therapy. A baseline

Box 29.1 Recommendations for Patients Taking Antiepileptic Drugs	
General recommendations for all patients	• Engage in daily regular weight-bearing physical activity (provided medically safe). • Maintain a balanced diet rich in protein, calcium, and vitamin D. • Stop smoking. • Minimize caffeine intake. • Minimize alcohol intake. • Take 1000 to 1500 mg of calcium (nutrition and supplement) daily • Take 1000 IU vitamin D supplement with non-enzyme, inducing AEDs and 2000 IU with enzyme-inducing AEDs daily.
Additional recommendations for patients with osteopenia or osteoporosis	• Follow all the general recommendations. • Take higher doses of vitamin D daily. • For osteoporosis, treat with an appropriate pharmaceutical agent to enhance bone formation (e.g., bisphosphonate). • Consult an endocrinologist.

From: Petty et al. (2005), Mintzer et al. (2006), Gissel et al. (2007), and Meier & Kraenzlin (2011).

dual-energy X-ray absorptiometry (DEXA) scan might be performed at the start of therapy for patients at significant risk for osteopenia or osteoporosis. Risks for decreased bone density include being nonambulatory or relatively inactive, institutionalized, or excessively thin. Postmenopausal women and patients with other medical risk factors such as concomitant steroid therapy are also at high risk. For patients not at risk, controversy exists over the value of a baseline DEXA scan, and one might wait until AED therapy has been taken for 5 years before performing this test. In children, some have recommended performing a DEXA scan even sooner, after 1 year of AED therapy in low-risk patients and after 6 months in high-risk patients (Kothare & Kaleyias, 2007). If there is evidence for decreased bone density on the DEXA scan, measure serum calcium, alkaline phosphatase, and 25-hydroxy vitamin-D levels and consider increasing doses of calcium and vitamin supplementation. Serial scans during the course of therapy are prudent and should be done every 1–3 years, depending on the results of the baseline DEXA scan, whether patients take agents presently known to cause osteoporosis or newer non-enzyme-inducing agents.

A recent systematic review and meta-analysis showed that, use of AEDs was associated with an 86% increase in the risk of fractures at any site, and a 90% increase in the risk of hip fractures. When the authors restricted the analysis to osteoporosis-related fractures, the risk remained higher, confirming the detrimental effect of AEDs on bone health. Among users of enzyme-inducing AEDs and users of non-enzyme-inducing AEDs, they found a significant difference in fracture risk, though the risks in both groups were higher compared with those in non-user controls (Shen et al., 2014).

A major issue relates to prescribing AEDs. For the patient who must be started on drug therapy, the higher potential for development of osteoporosis with enzyme-inducing AEDs provides an impetus to prescribe a newer, non-enzyme-inducing agent such as lamotrigine. This may cause less bone turnover and pose less risk for bone health. Should a patient presently take an enzyme-inducing drug or valproate, extra attention should be paid to bone health and calcium intake. In the absence of a problem, the commonsense measures advised above should be taken.

If a physician diagnoses osteoporosis or osteopenia in a patient who is presently taking an enzyme-inducing drug or valproate, what should be done? If the seizures are well controlled, there may be more risk of seizure recurrence if the AED is changed and patients may be reluctant to switch drugs. In that case, calcium and vitamin-D supplements should be prescribed at a minimum, in combination with a pharmaceutical agent to enhance bone formation (e.g., bisphosphonate) (Box 29.1). A follow-up DEXA scan should be performed in 1 year to assess response. If bone density is improved, then therapy does not need to be altered, and bone density can be monitored over the succeeding years. However, should these medical measures prove ineffective without improvement on subsequent bone density scans, then it is advisable to switch the patient to a non-enzyme-inducing AED.

References

Ali II, Schuh L, Barkley GL, Gates JR. Antiepileptic drugs and reduced bone mineral density. *Epilepsy and Behavior*. 2004;5: 296–300.

Babayigit A, Dirik E, Bober E, Cakmakci H. Adverse effects of antiepileptic drugs on bone mineral density. *Pediatric Neurology*. 2006;35: 177–181.

Beniczky SA, Viken J, Jensen LT, Andersen NB. Bone mineral density in adult patients treated with various antiepileptic drugs. *Seizure* 2012;21(6): 471–472.

Farhat G, Yamout B, Mikati MA, Demirjian S, Sawaya R, El-Hajj Fuleihan G. Effect of antiepileptic drugs on bone density in ambulatory patients. *Neurology*. 2002;58: 1348–1353.

Fekete S, Simko J, Gradosova I, Malakova J, Zivna H, Palicka V, Zivny P. The effect of levetiracetam on rat bone mass, structure and metabolism. *Epilepsy Res* 2013;107(1-2): 56–60.

Gissel T, Poulsen CS, Vestergaard P. Adverse effects of antiepileptic drugs on bone mineral density in children. *Expert Opinion in Drug Safety*. 2007;6: 267–278.

Koo DL, Joo EY, Kim D, Hong SB. Effects of levetiracetam as a monotherapy on bone mineral density and biochemical markers of bone metabolism in patients with epilepsy. *Epilepsy Res*. 2013;104(1–2): 134–139.

Koo DL, Hwang KJ, Han SW, Kim JY, Joo EY, Shin WC, Lee HW, Seo DW, Hong SB. Effect of oxcarbazepine on bone mineral density and biochemical markers of bone metabolism in patients with epilepsy. *Epilepsy Res*. 2014;108(3): 442–447.

Kothare SV, Kaleyias J. The adverse effects of antiepileptic drugs in children. *Expert Opinion in Drug Safety*, 2007;6:251–265.

Meier C, Kraenzlin ME. Antiepileptics and bone health. *Ther Adv Musculoskelet Dis*. 2011;3(5): 235–243.

Mintzer S, Boppana P, Toguri J, DeSantis A. Vitamin D levels and bone turnover in epilepsy patients taking carbamazepine or oxcarbazepine. *Epilepsia*. 2006;47: 510–515.

Pack AM, Morrell MJ, Marcus R, et al. Bone mass and turnover in women with epilepsy on antiepileptic drug monotherapy. *Annals of Neurology*. 2005;57: 252–257.

Petty SJ, Paton LM, O'Brien TJ, et al. Effect of antiepileptic medication on bone mineral measures. *Neurology*. 2005;65: 1358–1365.

Shen C, Chen F, Zhang Y, Guo Y, Ding M. Association between use of antiepileptic drugs and fracture risk: a systematic review and meta-analysis. *Bone*. 2014;64: 246–253.

Sheth RD, Hermann BP. Bone mineral density with lamotrigine monotherapy for epilepsy. *Pediatric Neurology*. 2007;37: 250–254.

Chapter 30

Antiepileptic Drugs in Patients With HIV Infection/AIDS

Central nervous system (CNS) complications occur in 39%–70% of patients with HIV/AIDS (Siddiqi & Birbeck, 2013). The incidence of seizures may be as high as 11% in HIV-infected patients (Liedtke et al., 2004; Kellinghaus et al., 2007). Etiology of seizures among patients with HIV/AIDS has a long list, including acute symptomatic (provoked) causes, central nervous system opportunistic infections, malignancy, stroke, dementia, and immune reconstitution inflammatory syndrome, among others. Though generalized seizures certainly exist in patients with HIV/AIDS, focal onset seizures are more likely due to the vulnerability of the CNS to brain lesions. Since provoked seizures are especially common among patients with HIV/AIDS, it is important to thoroughly evaluate the underlying cause for the seizure. A clinical assessment looking for sources of infection is needed and investigations should include serum glucose, sodium, calcium, magnesium, and creatinine; liver function tests, complete blood count, CD4 count, blood cultures, urine cultures, a toxicology screen, a chest X-ray, neuroimaging, and cerebrospinal fluid (CSF) examination. Electroencephalography (EEG) may be helpful in evaluating seizure recurrence risk and can distinguish encephalopathy from non-convulsive status epilepticus in patients with decreased level of consciousness (Siddiqi & Birbeck, 2013).

Although it is more common for patients with HIV/AIDS to subsequently develop epilepsy, people with epilepsy can certainly contract HIV. It is recommended to initiate antiretroviral drugs in all HIV-infected individuals, thus antiretroviral and antiepileptic (AED) co-administration is nearly unavoidable in this population. A discussion with the HIV physician is warranted. Ideally, an effective antiretroviral drug regimen with no clinically important drug interaction with the patient's established effective AED therapy will be selected. When this is not possible, a transition to another AED (discussed later) is needed. Recurrent seizures or increased seizure frequency should be evaluated more carefully in patients with epilepsy and HIV. One should maintain a low threshold for repeat neuroimaging and a lumbar puncture in a person with HIV and epilepsy to assure no underlying HIV-related pathology is contributing to seizure recurrence or exacerbation (Siddiqi & Birbeck, 2013).

When a patient with HIV/AIDS presents with an acute seizure, controlling the seizure is more important than concerns of compromising HIV therapy. Status epilepticus should be managed with standard protocol. After controlling an acute seizure, an evaluation must commence to assess the underlying etiology, risk of seizure recurrence and the need to start an AED. If seizure recurrence, abnormal imaging or abnormal EEG findings support chronic AED therapy, then careful consideration must be given to drug selection. The patient may need transition from the medication used acutely to something suitable for long-term use (Figure 30.1) (Siddiqi & Birbeck, 2013).

The combination regimens used to treat HIV infection often include substrates, inducers, and inhibitors of several cytochrome P-450 isoenzymes. Complex interactions may occur when some AEDs are administered to patients receiving treatment for HIV infection. The choice of an appropriate AED can therefore be challenging. For example, phenobarbital, phenytoin, and carbamazepine have complex drug-drug interactions and are suboptimal in these patients (Liedtke et al., 2004). In contrast, levetiracetam, lacosamide, gabapentin, and pregabalin are favorable AEDs to administer to patients with HIV/AIDS (Siddiqi & Birbeck, 2013). Although the choice of AED must consider efficacy against a seizure type or syndrome, it is equally important to address comorbid illnesses and comedications (Romanelli et al., 2000; Liedtke et al., 2004; Mullin et al., 2004).

Benzodiazepines

CYP3A4 inhibitors may reduce the metabolism of clonazepam and increase the potential for benzodiazepine toxicity. Examples of CYP3A4 inhibitors include some antiretroviral protease inhibitors (e.g., ritonavir) and non-nucleoside reverse transcriptase inhibitors (e.g., nevirapine) (Romanelli et al., 2000). Clobazam is similarly hepatically metabolized and may cause neurotoxicity from increased concentrations of clobazam when co-administered with the etravirine (Siddiqi & Birbeck, 2013).

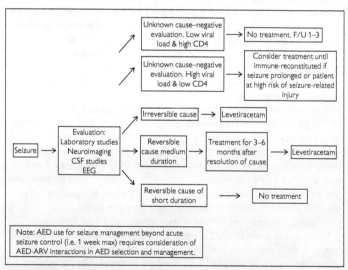

Figure 30.1 Algorithm for treatment of seizure in patients with HIV/AIDS.

AED: Antiepileptic drug; ARV: Antiretroviral; CSF: Cerebro-spinal fluid; EEG: Electroencephalography.

Adapted from: Siddiqi O, Birbeck GL. Safe Treatment of Seizures in the Setting of HIV/AIDS. *Curr Treat Options Neurol* 2013;15(4): 529–543.

Carbamazepine

Carbamazepine is suboptimal in HIV/AIDS patients because it is an enzyme inducer. Due to complex interactions, dose adjustments for carbamazepine and the antiretroviral medications may be needed. Both carbamazepine and antiretroviral medications are metabolized by cytochrome P-450 enzymes and can induce (carbamazepine) or inhibit (antiretroviral drugs) the cytochrome P-450 system.

Coadministration of ritonavir, a potent CYP3A4 inhibitor, and carbamazepine has resulted in increased carbamazepine concentrations and clinical toxicity (Garcia et al., 2000). Lopinavir/ritonavir and nelfinavir may decrease carbamazepine metabolism, causing an elevation in carbamazepine serum concentrations. Carbamazepine toxicity may be prevented by reducing the carbamazepine dosage by 25%–50% when protease inhibitors are introduced. A carbamazepine serum concentration should be repeated 3–5 days after the protease inhibitors are started (Bates & Herman, 2006). On the other hand, carbamazepine may increase the metabolism of the protease inhibitors, leading to decreased antiretroviral efficacy. The complexity of carbamazepine-PI interactions is amplified when two PIs are used in combination.

Coadministration of carbamazepine with non-nucleoside reverse transcriptase inhibitors results in complex interactions. For example, substantial reductions in delavirdine concentrations may occur. In addition, delavirdine may inhibit the metabolism of carbamazepine, resulting in increased carbamazepine concentrations (Romanelli et al., 2000).

If carbamazepine is used in patients being treated for HIV infection, the patient must be closely monitored for both antiviral efficacy and seizure control. If possible, a different AED should be used in HIV/AIDS patients.

Ethosuximide

Due to inhibitory effect of protease inhibitors on various hepatic isoenzymes, an interaction between ethosuximide and these drugs (e.g., delavirdine) may occur. This may necessitate up to a 50% dose reduction of ethosuximide. Non-nucleoside reverse transcriptase inhibitors may also have some clinically important drug interactions with ethosuximide (Romanelli et al., 2000). Closely monitor epilepsy patients during concurrent therapy.

Gabapentin

Gabapentin has no important interaction with antiretroviral drugs, has a favorable psychiatric profile, and is possibly helpful for HIV-associated neuropathies. Overall, gabapentin has a good profile for the treatment of seizures in HIV/AIDS patients (Romanelli et al., 2000; Mullin et al., 2004) and is a reasonable choice to treat seizures.

Lacosamide

Lacosamide is a good choice for treating seizures in patients with HIV. It has few, if any, drug interactions with antiretroviral drugs. However, adverse effects (e.g., dizziness, ataxia, syncope, and cardiac problems) may occur, and observation is warranted (Siddiqi & Birbeck, 2013).

Lamotrigine

Lamotrigine is a broad-spectrum AED that does not induce cytochrome P-450 enzymes. However, antiretroviral medications may affect lamotrigine plasma concentrations. Lopinavir/ritonavir and atazanovir/ritonavir both resulted in decreased bioavailability of lamotrigine when co-administered with lamotrigine. Therefore, careful therapeutic drug monitoring for lamotrigine may be required (Romanelli et al., 2000; Liedtke et al., 2004; Mullin et al., 2004; Siddiqi & Birbeck, 2013). Lamotrigine has a favorable cognitive and behavioral profile. This drug may be useful for HIV-associated neuropathies.

Levetiracetam

Levetiracetam is a broad-spectrum antiepileptic drug and is a good choice for treating seizures in patients with HIV. It has few, if any, drug interactions with antiretroviral drugs. However, behavioral and psychiatric adverse effects may occur, and observation is warranted (Mullin et al., 2004).

Oxcarbazepine

Oxcarbazepine probably has some drug interactions with antiretroviral drugs due to inhibition and induction of various hepatic enzymes (Liedtke et al., 2004). However, there is one report that showed that concurrent use of efavirenz and oxcarbazepine may not affect efavirenz plasma concentrations (Goicoechea et al., 2006). It should be used with caution in any patient with HIV/AIDS and hyponatremia as this may be further exacerbated with use of oxcarbazepine (Siddiqi & Birbeck, 2013). Oxcarbazepine has minimal cognitive side effects and may be efficacious in HIV-associated neuropathies (not studied in HIV patients but is efficacious in other neuropathic pains) (Mullin et al., 2004).

Perampanel

Data is not available with regard to interaction with antiretroviral drugs.

Phenobarbital/Primidone

These drugs are also suboptimal in patients with HIV. If phenobarbital (or primidone) is used in a patient being treated for HIV, the patient must be closely monitored for antiviral and barbiturate efficacy. Due to complex interactions, appropriate dose adjustments for phenobarbital or the anti-retroviral medications may be needed. Phenobarbital is an enzyme inducer and will likely increase the metabolism of some antiretroviral drugs, leading to decreased antiretroviral efficacy. Consequently, there is possibility for the development of resistant mutations of HIV. In addition, some protease inhibitors and non-nucleoside reverse transcriptase inhibitors may inhibit the metabolism of phenobarbital, resulting in increased phenobarbital concentrations (Romanelli et al., 2000; Mullin et al., 2004). If possible, a different AED should be used in HIV/AIDS patients.

Phenytoin

Complex interactions may occur when phenytoin or fosphenytoin is administered to patients receiving treatment for HIV infection, so these agents are suboptimal as well (unless, in patients with status epilepticus). If phenytoin is used in patients being treated for HIV infection, the patient must be closely monitored for antiviral efficacy and seizure control. Appropriate dose adjustments for phenytoin or the antiretroviral medications are not known. Phenytoin is an enzyme inducer and will likely increase the metabolism of some antiretroviral drugs, leading to decreased antiretroviral efficacy. It is recommended not to coadminister phenytoin with antiretroviral drugs due to the potential for subtherapeutic antiretroviral activity and the subsequent possibility for the development of resistant mutations of HIV. In addition, some protease inhibitors and non-nucleoside reverse transcriptase inhibitors may inhibit the metabolism of phenytoin, resulting in increased phenytoin concentrations and clinical toxicity. If possible, a different AED should be used in HIV/AIDS patients. However, if absolutely necessary (e.g., in patients with status epilepticus), phenytoin may be initiated and, to compensate for the enzyme-inducing effects of phenytoin, simultaneously increase antiretroviral medication dosage. Plasma levels of both phenytoin and antiretroviral drugs should be monitored (Romanelli et al., 2000; Mullin et al., 2004). If hypoalbuminemia is present, then free phenytoin levels should be measured (Romanelli et al., 2000).

Pregabalin

Pregabalin most likely has no important interactions with antiretroviral drugs, has a favorable psychiatric profile, and is possibly helpful for HIV-associated neuropathies. It is a reasonable choice in patients with HIV infection and seizure disorders.

Rufinamide

Rufinamide is hepatically metabolized. Therefore, it is not a first-line treatment candidate in patients with HIV/AIDS (Siddiqi & Birbeck, 2013).

Tiagabine

Tiagabine interacts with some antiretroviral drugs (e.g., efavirenz). This drug has significant adverse effects in the central nervous system. Tiagabine is not a favorable AED for the treatment of seizures in HIV/AIDS patients (Liedtke et al., 2004).

Topiramate

Topiramate is a broad-spectrum antiepileptic drug but may have complex interactions. Topiramate has interactions with some antiretroviral drugs (e.g., efavirenz) (Liedtke et al., 2004), and at dosages above 200 mg daily, it induces hepatic enzymes. Although not yet studied in HIV-associated neuropathy, it has been efficacious in other syndromes of neuropathic pain, including diabetic neuropathy. However, some patients may experience cognitive impairment, and thus it may not be a good AED for patients with AIDS-related dementia. Topiramate may be associated with weight loss, which is a consideration for patients with anorexia or generalized wasting. It has a mixed psychiatric profile (Mullin et al., 2004). It is therefore not a first choice to treat seizures in patients with HIV.

Valproate

Valproate has been associated with hepatic and multiorgan failure when used with antiretroviral drugs. In addition, valproate may have some interactions with antiretroviral drugs (e.g., zidovudine). Valproate is not a first choice in the treatment of epilepsy or other illnesses in patients with HIV/AIDS (Mullin et al., 2004).

Vigabatrin

Vigabatrin is usually reserved for patients with refractory epilepsy, when no other drug offers hope. The associated adverse side effects (i.e., vision loss) could be devastating (Siddiqi & Birbeck, 2013).

Zonisamide

Zonisamide is metabolized by hepatic cytochrome P-450 isoenzyme 3A4 (CYP3A4). Enzyme inhibitors can therefore increase the serum levels of zonisamide. Many drugs including antiretroviral protease inhibitors are known to inhibit the CYP3A4 isoenzyme (Romanelli et al., 2000). Serum levels should be monitored if these agents are used, and lower doses of zonisamide may be used. Because of interactions, this drug is not a first choice to treat seizures in patients with HIV infection.

Recommended Antiepileptic Drugs in Patients With HIV Infection/AIDS

1. **Generalized epilepsies:** Levetiracetam
2. **Focal epilepsies:** Gabapentin, lacosamide, levetiracetam, pregabalin.

References

Bates DE, Herman RJ. Carbamazepine toxicity induced by lopinavir/ritonavir and nelfinavir. *Annals of Pharmacotherapy*. 2006;40: 1190–1195.

Garcia AB, Ibarra AL, Etessam JP, et al. Protease inhibitor-induced carbamazepine toxicity. *Clinical Neuropharmacology*. 2000;23: 216–218.

Goicoechea M, Best B, Capparelli E, et al. Concurrent use of efavirenz and oxcarbazepine may not affect efavirenz plasma concentrations. *Clinical Infectious Disease*. 2006;43: 116–167.

Kellinghaus C, Engbring C, Kovac S, et al. Frequency of seizures and epilepsy in neurological HIV-infected patients. *Seizure*. 2008;17(1): 27–33.

Liedtke MD, Lockhart SM, Rathbun RC. Anticonvulsants and antiretroviral interactions. *Annals of Pharmacotherapy*. 2004;38: 482–489.

Mullin P, Green G, Bakshi R. Special populations: the management of seizures in HIV-positive patients. *Current Neurology and Neuroscience Reports*. 2004;4: 308–314.

Romanelli F, Jennings HR, Nath A, Ryan M, Berger J. Therapeutic dilemma: the use of anticonvulsants in HIV-positive individuals. *Neurology*. 2000;54: 1404–1407.

Siddiqi O, Birbeck GL. Safe Treatment of Seizures in the Setting of HIV/AIDS. *Curr Treat Options Neurol*. 2013;15(4): 529–543.

Index

Page numbers followed by *f* or *t* indicate figures or tables. Page numbers followed by *b* indicate boxes.